T0074165

Ralf Kiesslich

Peter R. Galle

Markus F. Neurath

Atlas of Endomicroscopy

Ralf Kiesslich

Peter R. Galle

Markus F. Neurath

Atlas of Endomicroscopy

With 156 Figures and 8 Tables

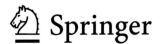 Springer

Prof. Dr. Ralf Kiesslich
Leiter der Interdisziplinären Endoskopie

Prof. Dr. Peter R. Galle
Direktor der I. Med. Klinik

Prof. Dr. Markus Neurath
Direktor des Instituts für Molekulare Medizin

I. Med. Clinic
Johannes Gutenberg University of Mainz
Langenbeckstr. 1
55131 Mainz, Germany

ISBN 978-3-540-34757-6 Springer Medizin Verlag Heidelberg

Bibliografische Information der Deutschen Bibliothek
The Deutsche Bibliothek lists this publication in Deutsche Nationalbibliographie;
detailed bibliographic data is available in the internet at http://dnb.ddb.de.

Springer Medizin Verlag
springer.com
© Springer Medizin Verlag Heidelberg 2008

SPIN 11768685
Typesetting: TypoStudio Tobias Schaedla, Heidelberg
Printing: Stürtz GmbH, Würzburg

18/5135/BK – 5 4 3 2 1 0

Prologue

Daniel K. Podolsky

Diseases of the gastrointestinal tract are many and varied, reflecting the complexities of structure and the processes that underlie normal digestive function. Over the past decades, our approaches to the evaluation of patients with gastrointestinal disorders and the study of their underlying processes have been transformed by the evolution of endoscopy. The history of modern gastrointestinal endoscopy began with the development of tools that allowed the direct inspection of mucosal surfaces, beginning with endoscopes that depended on incandescent light, pioneered by Schindler, and followed by the refinement possible through incorporation of fibre-optic technology and, more recently, use of the CCD chip. These have enabled progressively better visualisation of surface features. There also have been significant expansions of the usefulness of these scopes beyond en face visualisation, including the cannulation of biliary and pancreatic duct structures for radiological imaging and, most importantly, the development of interventional adjuncts beginning with mucosal biopsy and now encompassing many therapeutic devices.

We now find ourselves in an era in which scopes that enable access to endoluminal sites permit deeper types of analysis, figuratively and literally, of the gastrointestinal tract. This is well exemplified by endoscopic ultrasonography and more recently by optical coherence tomography. Confocal laser »endomicroscopy« (CLE) places the gastroenterologist at a new threshold. The cellular resolution possible allows the physician to directly evaluate, in life, histological structures that were previously the purview of only the pathologist in examining fixed tissue specimens. Much as the evolution of other endoscopic techniques has merged the skills of the gastroenterologist with imaging previously only within the realm of the radiologist, these techniques will require the gastroenterologist to become as finely attuned to microscopic structure as the pathologist in order to complement the familiarity with the surface appearances that have been the historical mainstay of endoscopy.

The true value of confocal laser endomicroscopy will emerge only with intensive characterisation that will build on the knowledge described in this volume. Delineation of the confocal laser endomicroscopic findings that are present across various digestive diseases is needed, and demonstration that knowledge of these microscopic features results in more precise diagnosis and prognosis beyond that possible through conventional endoscopy will be essential. It is incumbent on the GI community to ensure that the power of endomicroscopy is also applied to gain greater insight into normal mucosal function and disease processes, including response to therapy. Many technologies with apparent promise have ultimately failed to have a significant impact on clinical practice as their utility and limitations became more clear with experience. In that sense it must be said that the jury is still out for CLE. However, early experience, as described for the first time in this volume, has already yielded a remarkable amount of information about a technology that was virtually unknown just a few short years ago. These observations suggest that this approach indeed has great promise and will find an important place in gastroenterology. Clinicians and investigators both should embrace the opportunity and challenge provided by this powerful new means of visualising the gastrointestinal tract. This text is a milestone on the way to achieving these goals.

Foreword

Dear Reader,

Endomicroscopy is a newly developed diagnostic tool which enables in vivo microscopy with subcellular resolution during ongoing endoscopy. Thus, endomicroscopy is a revolutionary technology, providing endoscopists for the first time with information about living cells in human beings. Endoscopy and pathology are no longer separate subjects, and thus endomicroscopy leads to a close interaction between the endoscopist and the pathologist.

The *Atlas of Endomicroscopy* is the first book dealing with the new insights provided by endomicroscopy and gives an overview of the development, the requirements, the technique, the current indications and further possibilities of endomicroscopy.

This book was possible thanks to the excellent contributions of the various authors, all of whom are experts in their fields. We, as the editors, are deeply grateful for their contributions and visions.

Endomicroscopy today represents the beginning of a new era; further technical improvements and refinements are emerging and new diagnostic possibilities present themselves almost daily. It is absolutely worthwhile to learn about the new possibilities of endomicroscopy because it will influence our clinical algorithm now and in the future. Today, it is possible to analyse the mucosal architecture in vivo, which leads to targeted and safe mucosal biopsies. Tomorrow, new contrast agents might greatly facilitate the diagnosis of cancerous tissue with clear visualisation of distinct malignant epitopes (molecular imaging).

This atlas will provide you with the information necessary to begin using endomicroscopy in your own practice and will provide an understanding of its possibilities and current limitations. We hope that you will find it of great value for your daily work.

Creating and writing a book about a newly developing technique is always a challenge because things must be described for the first time. We received great help and support from many colleagues and we would like to acknowledge them. Kerry Dunbar, from Johns Hopkins University, helped in writing and editing the book. Katharina Lammersdorf, Bettina Müller and Marcus Kerner, students from Mainz University, helped substantially to develop a confocal database which simplified the identification of suitable images for the atlas. We also wish to acknowledge Professor Adrian Polglase and Professor Finlay Macrae of Cabrini Hospital for consenting to our use of clinical endomicroscopy images of the human colonic and small bowel mucosa (which were among the first ever obtained in human subjects in vivo). Finally, we thank Dr. Rupert Leong of Bankstown-Lidcombe Hospital in Sydney, Australia, for providing some imaging examples of coeliac disease.

Ralf Kiesslich
Peter R. Galle
Markus F. Neurath

Contents

List of Contributors

Editors

Prof. Dr. Ralf Kiesslich
Leiter der Interdisziplinären Endoskopie
Medizinische Klinik I
Johannes Gutenberg-Universität Mainz
Langenbeckstr. 1
D-55131 Mainz

Prof. Dr. Peter R. Galle
Direktor der I. Med. Klinik
Medizinische Klinik I
Johannes Gutenberg-Universität Mainz
Langenbeckstr. 1
D-55131 Mainz

Prof. Dr. Markus Neurath
Direktor des Instituts für Molekulare
Medizin
Medizinische Klinik I
Johannes Gutenberg-Universität Mainz
Langenbeckstr. 1
D-55131 Mainz

Authors

Dr. Raja Atreya
Medizinische Klinik I
Johannes Gutenberg-Universität Mainz
Langenbeckstr. 1
D-55131 Mainz

Dr. Christian Bojarski
Charité - CC10
Campus Benjamin Franklin
Zentrale Endoskopie
Hindenburgdamm 30
D-12203 Berlin

Marcia Irene Canto, M.D., M.H.S.
Johns Hopkins University
1830 E. Monument Street, Room 425
Baltimore, MD 21205
U.S.A.

Dr. Ralph S. DaCosta
Division of BioPhysics and BioImaging
University of Toronto
Ontario Cancer Institute / University
Health Network
610 University Avenue
Toronto, Ontario, M5G 2M9
Canada

Peter Delaney
Optiscan Pty, Ltd,
15-17 Normanby Rd
Notting Hill,
VIC 3168
Australia

Kerry Dunbar, M.D.
Johns Hopkins University
1830 E. Monument Street, Room 425
Baltimore, MD 21205
U.S.A.

Prof. Dr. Christian Ell
HSK Dr. Horst Schmidt Klinik
Zentrum Innere Medizin
Leiter der Klinik Innere Medizin II
Ludwig-Erhard-Str. 100
D-65199 Wiesbaden

Prof. Dr. Wolfgang Fischbach
Klinikum Aschaffenburg
Medizinische Klinik II
Chefarzt Gastroenterologie und
Enterologie
Am Hasenkopf
D-63739 Aschaffenburg

Dr. Martin Goetz
Medizinische Klinik I
Johannes Gutenberg-Universität Mainz
Langenbeckstr. 1
D-55131 Mainz

Dr. Arthur Hoffman
Medizinische Klinik I
Johannes Gutenberg-Universität Mainz
Langenbeckstr. 1
D-55131 Mainz

PD Dr. Jörg Carl Hoffmann
Freie Universität Berlin
Medizinische Klinik I
Gastroenterologie Infektiologie und
Rheumatologie
Hindenburgdamm 30
D-12203 Berlin

Dr. David P. Hurlstone
Royal Hallamshire Hospital,
Sheffield, UK
17 Alexandra Gardens
Lyndhurst Road
Nether Edge
Sheffield, S11 9DQ
U.K.

Dr. Tomohiro Kato, M.D., Ph.D.
Assistant professor
Division of Gastroenterology
and Hepatology
Department of Internal Medicine
The Jikei University School of Medicine
Nishi-shinbashi 3-25-8
Minato-ku,Tokyo 1058461
Japan

Dr. Christoph Loddenkemper
Charité - Universitätsmedizin Berlin
Charité Campus Benjamin Franklin
Institut für Pathologie
Hindenburgdamm 30
D-12203 Berlin

Dr. Norman E. Marcon
St. Michael's Hospital
Center for Therapeutic Endoscopy &
Endoscopic Oncology
16-062 Victoria Wing
30 Bond Street
Toronto, Ontario, M5B 1W8
Canada

Wendy McLaren, Ph.D.
Optiscan Pty, Ltd,
15-17 Normanby Rd
Notting Hill,
VIC 3168
Australia

Dr. Marshall Montrose
Dept of Molecular & Cellular
Physiology
University of Cincinnati
231 Albert Sabin Way
Cincinnati OH 45267-0576
U.S.A.

Prof. Dr. Horst Neuhaus
Chefarzt der Medizinischen Klinik
Evangelisches Krankenhaus
Kirchfeldstraße 40
D-40217 Düsseldorf

Dr. Oliver Pech
HSK Dr. Horst Schmidt Klinik
Zentrum Innere Medizin
Klinik Innere Medizin II
Ludwig-Erhard-Str. 100
D-65199 Wiesbaden

Daniel K. Podolsky, MD
Chief, Gastrointestinal Unit
Massachusetts General Hospital
Blake 4
55 Fruit St.
Boston, MA 02114
U.S.A.

Prof. Dr. Harald Stein
Charité - Universitätsmedizin Berlin
Charité Campus Benjamin Franklin
Direktor des Institutes für Pathologie
Hindenburgdamm 30
D-12203 Berlin

Steven Thomas, Ph.D.
Optiscan Pty, Ltd,
15-17 Normanby Rd
Notting Hill,
VIC 3168
Australia

PD Dr. med. Michael Vieth
Institut für Pathologie
Klinikum Bayreuth
Preuschwitzer Straße 101
D-95445 Bayreuth

**Prof. Dr. Alastair J.M. Watson M.D.
F.R.C.P.**
School of Clinical Sciences
The Henry Wellcome Laboratory
Nuffield Building
University of Liverpool
Crown St.
Liverpool. L69 3GE
U.K.

Dr. Brian C. Wilson
Division of BioPhysics and BioImaging
University of Toronto
Ontario Cancer Institute / University
Health Network
610 University Avenue
Toronto, Ontario, M5G 2M9
Canada

Dr. med. Katja Wirths
Evangelisches Krankenhaus Düsseldorf
Kirchfeldstraße 40
D-40217 Düsseldorf

Prof. Dr. Martin Zeitz
Charité - CC10
Campus Benjamin Franklin
Zentrale Endoskopie
Hindenburgdamm 30
D-12203 Berlin

Development of Endoscopic Devices: Past, Present and Future

Norman E. Marcon, Brian C. Wilson, Ralph S. DaCosta

Key concepts:
- CCD equipped white light video endoscopy is currently considered state of the art for endoscopy of the GI-tract
- Confocal laser endoscopy (CLE) currently provides the best in situ histology quality imaging.

1.1 Introduction

The application of fibre optics beginning 40 years ago was revolutionary in allowing us to access and assess the gastrointestinal tract, and we have not looked back since. In the early days of modern endoscopy the emphasis was placed primarily on patients with symptoms, or on the diagnosis and biopsy of lesions first seen or suspected with barium contrast imaging. Progress in instrument design, driven by clinical need, and technological advancements in device development have enabled brighter illumination of the tissue surface, improved endoscopic image contrast and the capturing and transmission of higher resolution images, thus providing endoscopists with a clearer and more robust visualisation of the mucosal field. This, in turn, has facilitated the detection of smaller and more subtle dysplastic lesions. The implementation of various dye-spraying contrast agents (i.e. absorbed and non-absorbed) applied topically to the luminal surface during endoscopic procedures has also contributed to the improved detection of dysplasia.

An illustrative example of the application of fibre-optic endoscopy is the pioneering work of Japanese endoscopists in the field of upper GI cancers. They recognised the public health impact of their most common malignancy and, in conjunction with industry, developed gastrocameras and endoscopes to enhance the early detection, diagnosis and staging of gastric cancers. This led to a national mass screening program. These changes resulted in a clear reduction in the rate of gastric cancer. In Japan, 50% of gastric cancers are now diagnosed at an early stage and are curable by either endoscopic or surgical means [1, 2]. This large-volume screening has benefited endoscopists everywhere by bringing to our attention the need to examine the mucosa more carefully and to always be looking for early, subtle dysplastic lesions. However, in the Western world, although the incidence is much lower, only 5–10% of such gastric lesions are diagnosed at an early stage [3]. It has been suggested that this inconsistency might be partially related to the fact that Western endoscopists are less observant of subtle mucosal abnormalities. This difference between Japanese and Western endoscopists was crisply termed by Dr. Rene Lambert the 'eyes wide shut' concept [4]. Although scolding, this opinion raises the possibility that it is the smaller and more troublesome subtle dysplastic lesions that present the greatest challenge for the endoscopist. The identification of obvious large lesions is no longer a challenge, but with the increasing emphasis on endoscopic therapy and minimally invasive surgery, the search continues for improved endoscopic detection. Furthermore, the role of potential biomarkers to better select patients for endoscopic surveillance and monitoring may have more economic and clinical impact on screening for malignancy. Hopefully, the addition of new optical technologies, such as autofluorescence-based endoscopy, fluorescence endoscopy, narrow band imaging, optical coherence tomography and confocal laser endomicroscopy (CLE) will help all endoscopists to excel in this new field of endoscopic oncology.

In the context of this introductory chapter, in which we address the past, present and future of endoscopic device development, we use the term 'present' to define those endoscopic techniques that are in routine clinical practice and not those prototype devices that are currently being evaluated in endoscopic centres of excellence. Furthermore, more accurately we consider the present to include the 'state-of-the-art' in endoscopic practice since 2005. However, the authors concede that the state-of-the-art is a 'moving target', often determined by opinion leaders, centres of excellence, the need to publish and commercial pressures which are already driving the next generation of endoscopic devices.

1.2   The Present

Early detection of cancers at the stage of dysplasia has always been the dream of endoscopists. When endoscopy was first developed and employed clinically, its main application was in the diagnosis of symptomatic patients. The role of endoscopy was to confirm or exclude a diagnosis that was suspected on clinical grounds (e.g. dysphagia, anaemia, bleeding) or on the basis of radiological barium studies. However, its role in screening or surveillance is a more recent development in the West. The need and the capacity to screen large populations of asymptomatic individuals in a manner that is cost-effective and also improves outcome pose a dilemma that involves not only health care professionals but also governmental funding agencies.

Ideally, the selection of asymptomatic patients for endoscopy would be based on a biomarker present in urine, blood or stool that would better select the population to be investigated by screening endoscopy and that would have a greater likelihood of benefiting from a therapeutic intervention if a dysplastic lesion were found. However, such a technology is not likely to become available in the near future. Therefore, we will continue to rely on endoscopic assessment. In colonoscopy, aside from the prerequisites of a superb bowel-prep, careful visualisation and measured withdrawal time, the endoscopist using conventional white-light endoscopes should be able to recognise most lesions greater than 5 mm. However, flat lesions are notoriously difficult to recognise even for an observant endoscopist. Dye-spraying to detect subtle flat lesions, and their subsequent histological classification based on pit-patterns visualised by magnification endoscopy, is more commonly used in Japan [5] but is not in regular practice in North America or Europe.

The ability to determine whether a colonic polyp is adenomatous or hyperplastic and whether it need be excised is typically influenced by its size, colour, shape, boundary, consistency, and by whether it is liftable with a submucosal injection of saline [6]. Yet some may argue that this histological differentiation between benign and dysplastic polyps during endoscopy, at least in the non-diseased colon, is superfluous, as the lesion is likely to be removed and retrieved in either case [7]. However, in at-risk patients with field defects, such as with Barrett's oesophagus or ulcerative colitis, the issue of real-time histological characterisation and mapping is more crucial [8]. We speculate that better mapping of dysplasia and, ideally, real-time histology would greatly influence management of these patients.

Detection of early dysplastic lesions in the GI tract is essential for cure, because prognosis and ultimate survival are related to the size and stage of the lesion (i.e. mural invasiveness and positive node status). Additionally, outcomes such as survival and quality of life would be significantly enhanced by administering treatment while the lesion remains confined to the mucosa. Screening colonoscopy has demonstrated a long-term risk reduction in asymptomatic individuals [9]. An illustrative example is The National Polyp Study in the United States, which demonstrated a significant reduction in the incidence of colon cancer ranging from 76% to 90% as a result of polypectomy [10]. Although impressive at the time, these results remain suboptimal [11]. Why reduction was not closer to 100% might be related to the fact that diminutive lesions may have been missed for several reasons, including an inadequately prepared bowel, a poor endoscopic technique with incomplete polyp removal, or an inexperienced eye for subtle mucosal lesions. This emphasises the importance of improving existing endoscopic techniques in the recognition of subtle abnormalities. Further, the detection of early intraepithelial neoplasia in the GI tract in the properly selected patient with a well-staged lesion confined to the mucosa can allow curative endoscopic resection or ablation but will require long-term endoscopic surveillance. However, surgical resection is mandated for patients found to have multifocal disease or locally advanced disease not suitable for conventional endoscopic therapy.

For today's endoscopist, imaging of the gastrointestinal tract is best done using CCD-equipped white-light video endoscopy. This new technology provides clear high-resolution images of the mucosal lining and is now considered state of the art. There continues to be improvement in resolution as the chip-based technology gallops forward with higher pixel densities and miniaturisation. This application of chip technology is part of modern life and is largely related to the commercialisation of every conceivable type of imaging device, ranging from digital cameras to camera-equipped cellular telephones. Endoscopes with magnifying capabilities have been commonly used in Japan, but only in the past decade has there been interest and recognition of their usefulness in the West. The magnifying capability of these devices is best utilised once a suspicious lesion has been identified by wide-field scanning. In a featureless flat surface without 'obvious' irregularities the endoscopist needs a 'red flag' or 'waving hand' technique such as dye spraying, narrow band imaging or autofluorescence to determine the presence of occult dysplasia by identifying suspicious areas requiring further examination.

1.3 The Future

Ultimately, what the 'lazy endoscopist' desires is a technology that allows him to scan a wide area of mucosa combined with the capability to identify suspect lesions without having to spend a lot of time using the 'woodpecker' technique of multiple biopsies (i.e. the waving hand or red flag). In other words, we desire an imaging system that tells us where to focus our eye and allows us to obtain a spatial map of dysplastic lesions.

The candidates for this 'red flag' or 'waving hand' technology include autofluorescence imaging, narrow band imaging (NBI), and chromoendoscopy with dye spraying, all of which satisfy the clinical need to survey a large area of tissue. As an attempt to eliminate the need for messy dyes, NBI has been shown in Barrett's oesophagus to be equal to the use of high-resolution endoscopy plus indigo-carmine dye spraying [12]. NBI is a new technology based on a sim-

ple concept of spectral imaging (akin to 'electronic chromoendoscopy'). Although NBI features which are currently available in Olympus and Fujinon production models have caught the imagination of endoscopists, these devices are only now entering clinical use and their dissemination is still limited to a few academic centres and community hospitals. Considerable research remains to be done in several centres aside from the two or three leaders who have published already [12, 13]. For NBI, the Olympus NBI system is literally one blue band, while other technologies, such as the Fujinon Intelligent Chromoendoscopy (FICE) system, have several bands to choose from. Their application is related to the concept that perhaps different tissues are optimally scanned with different wavelengths (i.e. squamous, Barrett's, gastric, biliary and colonic mucosa). This is a fertile area for research in the coming years. Ultimately, determining the clinical role of NBI will require rigorous clinical evaluation in large-scale trials.

Autofluorescence imaging has been under clinical evaluation for almost 15 years and its role is yet to be defined. Our own studies have recently shown that in the colon autofluorescence imaging can improve the detection of diminutive adenomas by 19% and that it improves the differentiation between hyperplastic and dysplastic polyps by 20%, compared with conventional white light [14]. Recent studies suggest that autofluorescence imaging will have a positive impact on the detection of high-grade dysplasia in Barrett's oesophagus [15]. Additionally, new research investigating the concept of fluorescence-based tissue-specific contrast agents (i.e. fluorescent dye or quantum dot bioconjugate probes) has shown promise in animal models of upper and lower GI-tract cancers by causing suspicious precancerous lesions to light up [16, 17].

If the 'waving hand' beckoned like a glowing beacon, then the endoscopist traditionally would subject the area to excisional biopsies with forceps or the endoscopic mucosal resection (EMR) technique. However, there seems to be great promise in the concept of a so-called optical biopsy which would allow real-time in situ histology, comparable to what a pathologist would see with standard ex vivo H&E-stained tissue microscopy. Such a capability would enable real-time, almost instantaneous diagnosis with precise mapping of lesion boundaries, and it might be expected that the basal aspects of excision could be monitored at the same time. Examples of optical biopsy techniques include optical coherence tomography (OCT) [18], endocytoscopy [19], and confocal laser endomicroscopy (CLE) [20]. In its current

1

form, endocytoscopy (■ Fig. 1.1) is indeed surface imaging (e.g. approximately 25 µm deep). CLE, on the other hand, can supply tomographically reconstructed images with subcellular resolution to a depth of about 250 µm. OCT (■ Fig. 1.2) would theoretically be the closest to an optimal imaging device because light penetration may be as deep as 1500–2000 µm. However, the challenge to produce high-resolution »H&E-grade« OCT images has not yet been met.

The technology that has currently undergone the most evaluation and is closest to clinical acceptance and utility is the confocal laser endomicroscope. This highly focused probe allows reconstructed tomographic images down to a tissue depth of 250 µm. It permits direct observation of pathological tissue changes at the microscopic level, rather than traditional inference based on indirect changes at the macroscopic level. The images currently published are comparable to H&E-grade histology. Other applications of

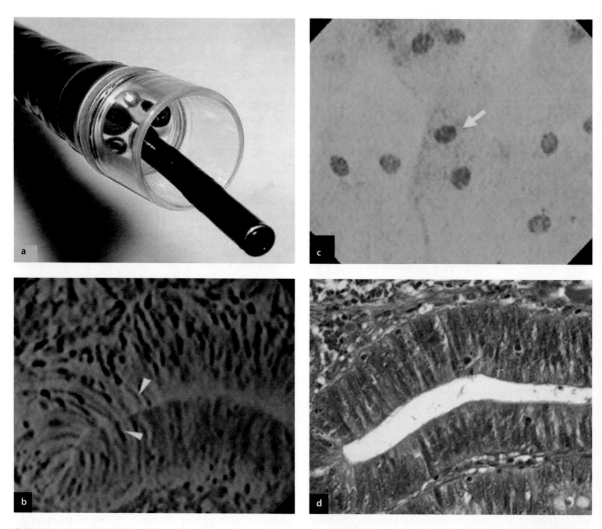

■ **Fig. 1.1a–d.** Endocytoscopy. **a** The endocytoscope is passed over the working channel of a standard endoscope (*arrow*) (with friendly permission of the author Y. Kumagai). A distal plastic cap is attached to the endoscope to reduce motion artefacts. **b** Single nuclei can be observed in the distal oesophagus after staining with methylene blue. **c** Single cells and in vivo architecture can also be observed in the colon. Here, an adenoma is displayed. The nuclei are enlarged and thickened, leading to the diagnosis of a tubular adenoma with low-grade dysplasia. **d** Corresponding histology (Reprinted from Gastrointestinal Endoscopy 63 (7), K. Sasajima et al., Real-time in vivo virtual histology of colorectal lesions when using the endocytoscopy system. 1010-1017. 2006. with permission from Elsevier)

this high-resolution imaging could allow the immediate examination of the 'EMR defect' to evaluate its lateral and basal margins for residual dysplasia. Also, with further miniaturisation, this technique could be applied to the biliary and pancreatic ducts and perhaps to fine-needle aspiration punctures in the assessment of extramucosal masses and pancreatic cystic lesions. Furthermore, fluorescence contrast agents may also enhance the utility of confocal fluorescence microendoscopy by providing functional and molecular information at the cellular level in vivo [17].

This 'knock-your-socks off' imaging technology does inadvertently pose some important unresolved issues for the endoscopist. For instance, in the early learning curve, having a pathologist at the endoscopist's side may well be mandatory. Currently, as investigators continue to evaluate where this technology fits into the diagnostic algorithm, there is a good opportunity to bring the GI pathologist into the endoscopy unit rather than having him sitting at a remote microscope and examining biopsies obtained days previously. As the technology becomes more acceptable and widespread, we can foresee that suitably trained endoscopists should be able to interpret this histology without the hand-holding of the pathologist.

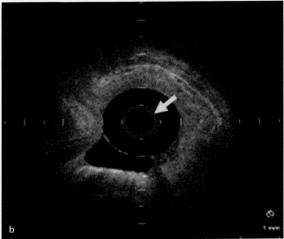
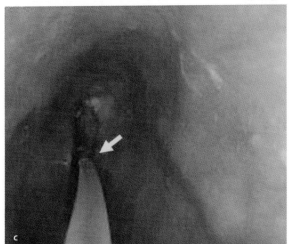
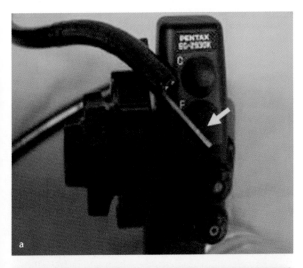
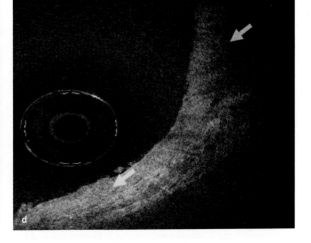

☐ **Fig. 1.2a–d.** Optical coherence tomography. **a** The OCT probe can be passed over the working channel of a conventional endoscope. **b** Light is used to analyse overall microarchitecture. **c** The probe is centred (*arrow*) in the middle of the oesophageal lumen. **d** Squamous epithelium (*lower arrow*) can be differentiated from squamous epithelium (*upper arrow*) due to different light patterns

Although confocal laser endomicroscopy is a phenomenal breakthrough, as it currently provides the best in situ histology-quality imaging, white-light endoscopy will continue to be fundamental to clinical practice. However, we speculate that in the not too distant future confocal endomicroscopy will become part of an endoscopic platform that will provide diagnostic mapping, staging and monitoring of therapy and therapeutic response in addition to exquisite histological-grade images in vivo – the 'superscope'.

References

1. Shimizu S, Tada M, Kawai K (1995) Early gastric cancer: its surveillance and natural course. Endoscopy. 27:27–31
2. Ikeda Y, Mori M, Koyanagi N, Wada H, Hayashi H, Tsugawa K, Miyazaki M, Haraguchi Y, Sugimachi K (1998) Features of early gastric cancer detected by modern diagnostic technique. J Clin Gastroenterol. 27:60–62
3. Everett SM, Axon AT (1997) Early gastric cancer in Europe. Gut. 41:142–150
4. Lambert R, Jeannerod M, Rey JF (2004) Eyes wide shut. Endoscopy. 36:723–725
5. Kudo S, Rubio CA, Teixeira CR, Kashida H, Kogure E (2001) Pit pattern in colorectal neoplasia: endoscopic magnifying view. Endoscopy. 33:367–373
6. Kudo S, Tamegai Y, Yamano H, Imai Y, Kogure E, Kashida H (2001) Endoscopic mucosal resection of the colon: the Japanese technique. Gastrointest Endosc Clin N Am. 11:519–535
7. Paris Workshop on Columnar Metaplasia in the Esophagus and the Esophagogastric Junction, Paris, France, December 11–12, 2004. (2005) Endoscopy. 37:879–920
8. Kiesslich R, Fritsch J, Holtmann M, Koehler HH, Stolte M, Kanzler S, Nafe B, Jung M, Galle PR, Neurath MF (2003) Methylene blue-aided chromoendoscopy for the detection of intraepithelial neoplasia and colon cancer in ulcerative colitis. Gastroenterology. 124:880–888
9. Lieberman DA, Prindiville S, Weiss DG, Willett W; VA Cooperative Study Group 380 (2003) Risk factors for advanced colonic neoplasia and hyperplastic polyps in asymptomatic individuals. JAMA. 290:2959–2967
10. Winawer SJ, Zauber AG, Ho MN, O'Brien MJ, Gottlieb LS, Sternberg SS, Waye JD, Schapiro M, Bond JH, Panish JF, et al (1993) Prevention of colorectal cancer by colonoscopic polypectomy. The National Polyp Study Workgroup. N Engl J Med. 329:1977–1981
11. Bressler B, Paszat LF, Vinden C, Li C, He J, Rabeneck L (2004) Colonoscopic miss rates for right-sided colon cancer: a population-based analysis. Gastroenterology. 127:452–456
12. Kara MA, Peters FP, Rosmolen WD, Krishnadath KK, ten Kate FJ, Fockens P, Bergman JJ (2005) High-resolution endoscopy plus chromoendoscopy or narrow-band imaging in Barrett's esophagus: a prospective randomized crossover study. Endoscopy. 37:929–936
13. Sharma P, Bansal A, Mathur S, Wani S, Cherian R, McGregor D, Higbee A, Hall S, Weston A. (2006) The utility of a novel narrow band imaging endoscopy system in patients with Barrett's esophagus. Gastrointest Endosc 64:167–175
14. Zanati S, Marcon NE, Cirocco M, et al (2005) Onco-life fluorescence imaging during colonoscopy assists in the differentiation of adenomatous and hyperplastic polyps and improves detection rate of dysplastic lesions in the colon. Gastroenterology 128:A27–28
15. Kara MA, Peters FP, Ten Kate FJ, Van Deventer SJ, Fockens P, Bergman JJ. (2005) Endoscopic video autofluorescence imaging may improve the detection of early neoplasia in patients with Barrett's esophagus. Gastrointest Endosc 61:679–685
16. DaCosta RS, Wilson BC, Marcon NE (2000) Light-induced fluorescence endoscopy of the gastrointestinal tract. Gastrointest Endosc Clin N Am 10:37–69
17. DaCosta RS, Tang Y, Kalliomaki T, Reilly RM, Weersink R, Elford A, Marcon NE, Wilson BC (2002) In vitro, in vivo and ex vivo near-infrared fluorescence imaging of human colon adenocarcinoma by specific immunotargeting of a tumor-associated mucin in a xenograft mouse model. Gastroenterology 122 (4): 260 [Suppl. 1]
18. Evans JA, Nishioka NS (2005) The use of optical coherence tomography in screening and surveillance of Barrett's esophagus. Clin Gastroenterol Hepatol. 3 [Suppl 1]:S8–11
19. Inoue H, Kazawa T, Sato Y, Satodate H, Sasajima K, Kudo SE, Shiokawa A. (2004) In vivo observation of living cancer cells in the esophagus, stomach, and colon using catheter-type contact endoscope, »Endo-Cytoscopy system«. Gastrointest Endosc Clin N Am 14:589–594, x–xi
20. Kiesslich R, Goetz M, Vieth M, Galle PR, Neurath MF. (2005) Confocal laser endomicroscopy. Gastrointest Endosc Clin N Am 15:715–731 (review)

Surface Analysis with Magnifying Chromoendoscopy in the Colon

David P. Hurlstone

Key concepts:
- Colonic chromoscopy and magnifying chromoendoscopy are useful tools for discriminating neoplastic and non-neoplastic colorectal lesions.
- Both techniques require structured training and are not 100% sensitive or specific.
- Confocal laser endomicroscopy might further refine the characterisation of colonic lesions because it provides in vivo histology.

2.1 Background

The secondary prevention of colorectal cancer (CRC) assumes that early detection and resection of precursor lesions will disrupt the adenoma-carcinoma sequence and halt progression to invasive neoplastic disease. The adenoma-carcinoma sequence described by Morson has until now formed the rationale for endoscopic therapies directed at reducing the incidence of colorectal cancer. The fact that snare polypectomy of exophytic lesions (Paris class Ip/s) [1] fails to prevent progression to carcinoma in up to 24% of lesions [2] has prompted many authors to re-evaluate the prevalence and clinicopathological significance of flat and depressed (Paris 0–II / 0–IIa/c / 0–IIc/a) colorectal lesions in Western cohorts. Such lesions (see Paris classification, ◘ Table 2.1), although well described by the Japanese, have only recently been reported in Western cohorts [2]. Controversy has existed regarding their prevalence, anatomical localisation and histopathological characteristics. We recently reported in a large prospective study in the UK that Paris class 0–II morphology accounted for 38% of all lesions, where 82% of Paris 0–II lesions with high-grade dysplasia (HGD) and 90% of all Paris class 0–IIc were located in the right colon [2]. These data support similar trends reported in other series and stress the importance of detection and definitive endoscopic therapy, particularly given the imminent introduction of a nationwide CRC screening programme in the UK and other European countries [2].

Magnifying chromoendoscopy permits the in vivo examination of the colorectal surface crypt or pit pattern, which has a high correlation with stereomicroscopic appearances of resected specimens [3]. The premise of this technology is to provide surface analysis of colorectal lesions that can be used at the time of colonoscopy to enhance diagnostic precision and guide subsequent therapeutic strategies.

Regarding Paris class Ip/s lesions, magnifying chromoendoscopy is not required, as there is an established and validated correlation between size and neoplastic risk, which is the major consideration when choosing endoscopic snare polypectomy or surgical resection. However, Paris 0–II lesions do not conform to this basic rationale, where therapeutic decisions are highly dependent on the detailed morphological appearance, including the surface crypt architecture. Indeed, some authors propose that such lesions may favour a de novo pathogenic pathway where early submucosal invasion and risk of associated lymph node metastasis (LNM) can occur [2].

However, conflicting data concerning the sensitivity, specificity and overall accuracy of magnifying chromoendoscopy have become apparent in the setting of routine clinical practice [4–6]. Variability in these data is multifactorial, being in part related to operator experience [4, 5], chromoscopic technique and East-West ambiguity in morphological and histopathological classification [1].

2.2 Classification of Superficial Neoplastic Colorectal Neoplasia – a Consensus Workshop Approach

Following the adoption of the modified Vienna histopathological classification for intramucosal neoplasia by Eastern and Western pathologists in the year 2000, there is now a clear histopathological consensus regarding three major groups for intraepithelial neoplasia (IN); non-invasive low-grade dysplasia (LGD), non-invasive high-grade dysplasia (HGD) and invasive cancer (laminal invasion) [7]. However, to optimise the full potential benefits of the modified Vienna classification and continue to extrapolate clinically meaningful data, it was felt that the merging of endoscopic morphological terminology between East and West would be needed. To this end, the Paris Workshop consensus guidelines were published in 2002 and now form a practical morphological framework for all endoscopists (◘ Table 2.1) [1].

Detailed morphological assessment of a lesion at endoscopy is derived from both quantitative and qualitative criteria, including documentation of size and anatomical location. Morphological assessment requires the localised application of a contrast chromoscopic agent, which in the colorectum is usually indigo carmine (IC) 0.1–0.5% solution or methylene blue (MB) 0.1% locally applied to the lesion using the syringe push technique or via a trans-portal diffusion catheter [2]. At this stage in morphological grading, it is important that the macroscopic classification is determined only from the gross appearance. The initial macroscopic classification should not be influenced by adjunctive clinical information or supplementary histopathological findings (i.e. a demonstrable lesion of type 0 morphology may subsequently be 'up-staged' to an advanced neoplasm at histopathology using the p-TNM classification or, in the reverse situation, a lesion may be down-staged). Hence, in most Japanese studies, superficial lesions are classified according to sub-types of type 0 morphology that can be sub-grouped

◘ Table 2.1. The Paris classification of endoscopic lesion morphology

Endoscopic appearance	Paris class		Description
Protruded lesions	Ip		Pedunculated polyps
	Ips		Subpedunculated polyps
	Is		Sessile polyps
Flat elevated lesions	IIa		Flat elevation of mucosa
	IIa / IIc		Flat elevation with central depression
Flat lesions	IIb		Flat mucosal change
	IIc		Mucosal depression
	IIc / IIa		Mucosal depression with raised edge

into three distinct types: 0–I, polypoid; 0–II, non-polypoid and non-excavated; and 0–III, non-polypoid with a frank ulcer. Group I can again be divided to include type 0–Ip (pedunculated) and 0-Is (subpedunculated). Also, type 0-II lesions include three distinct subgroups: 0–IIa, elevated; 0–IIb, completely flat with the mucosa; and 0–IIc, slightly depressed without an ulcer crater. A depressed lesion with central depression is classified as a type 0–IIc+IIa in contrast to a primary elevated lesion with a central depression at its apex, 0–IIa+IIc – in the latter class the relative depression as a rule does not extend below the level of the adjacent normal mucosa. Such morphological differentiation, although complex, is of utmost importance clinically, as type 0–IIa+IIc lesions have a poor prognosis with an increased risk of deep submucosal invasion, LNM and associated lymphovenous involvement, and mucinous and/or poorly differentiated histopathological features [8]. Hence, detailed chromo-

◻ **Table 2.2.** Modified Kudo criteria for the classification of colorectal crypt architecture in vivo using high-magnification chromoscopic colonoscopy

Pit type	Characteristics	Appearance using magnifying chromoendoscopy	Pit size (mm)
I	Normal round pits		0.07+/- 0.02 mm
II	Stellate or papillary		0.09 +/- 0.02 mm
IIIs	Tubular / round pits Smaller than pit type I		0.03 +/- 0.01 mm
IIIL	Tubular / large		0.22+/- 0.09 mm
IV	Sulcus / gyrus		0.93 +/- 0.32 mm
V(a)	Irregular arrangement and sizes of IIIL, IIIs, IV type pit		N/A

scopic morphological assessment at index endoscopy is mandatory in guiding the most appropriate and safe endoluminal management complemented by magnifying chromoendoscopy crypt architecture analysis (pit pattern classification, ◻ Table 2.2).

2.3 Stereomicroscopy and 'Pit Patterns' in the Human Colon

Topologically, the lumens of crypts show various shapes, subsequently grouped into five categories by Kudo, each predicting histological alterations [3]. The same features can be observed at the mucosal surface using a magnifying colonoscope.

2.4 Pit-pattern Classification and Magnification-Chromoscopic Appearances

Establishment of the neoplastic characteristics, including the potential for deep submucosal invasion, using stereomicroscopy is a well-established histopathological practice. Kosaka first reported the stereomicroscopic observation of the pit pattern in Paris class Ip/s lesions [9]. Subsequently, Nishizawa reported stereomicroscopic findings of minute, early superficial neoplasms describing the absence of glandular orifices or non-structural pit patterns [10]. Kudo later conducted stereomicroscopic observations in approximately 1600 lesions, enabling the creation of the established pit classification now used in Japanese and European colonoscopic practice. Kudo validated pit-pattern comparison between stereomicroscopic chromoscopy and magnification video-chromoscopy in 2001 [3]. These data demonstrated a high correlation rate between in vivo magnification chromoscopy as compared with ex vivo stereomicroscopy. Within the Kudo class, five types of pit pattern are described according to macroscopic morphology and size (◻ Table 2.2).

2.5 Magnification Chromoscopy in Routine Clinical Practice

The techniques of chromoendoscopy and magnification colonoscopy are potentially powerful tools for the detection and characterisation of Paris class II colorectal lesions. Detection of advanced colorectal neoplasia and large Paris class I lesions does not require chromoscopic enhancement [2]. However, in a manner similar to Paris class 0–II colorectal lesions, pit-pattern appearances at the surface in Paris class Is/p lesions can help predict neoplastic invasive depth [11]. 'On-table' management of such lesions may change radically with the use of pit-pattern classification. For example, management may include attempted endoscopic resection, 'guided' biopsies, and tattooing or endoclip marking for later surgical intervention.

Often subtle endoscopic signs such as mucosal erythema, paleness, haemorrhagic spots, absence of vascular network pattern, unevenness or mucosal deformity initially point to Paris type 0–II colorectal lesions [2]. It is following detection of such mucosal abnormalities that magnifying chromoendoscopy becomes a useful tool.

Qualitative diagnosis of early cancer is often reflected by endoscopic features of marginal irregularity, a 'star-shaped' depression, air-induced deformation (under altered air volume) and the absence of innominate grooves [2]. Such endoscopic abnormalities should prompt localised chromoscopy to augment accurate morphological classification of the lesion. Subsequent magnifying views can determine abnormal pit-pattern structure; particularly pit types IIIs and V (Vn), which may signify overt neoplastic change with deep invasive mucosal characteristics and hence associated LNM [2].

2.6 Current Endoluminal In Vivo Imaging Techniques

2.6.1 Limitations and Data Summary

In 1993, the Olympus 200Z series colonoscope was introduced, which permitted in vivo magnification of up to 100x normal. Using magnifying chromoendoscopy it is therefore possible to examine the detailed morphology and colonic pit or crypt patterns previously described using ex vivo stereomicroscopy [3]. The premise of this technology is to provide surface crypt analysis that can be used at the time of colonoscopy to enhance diagnostic precision and help guide subsequent therapeutic strategies. Such strategies are highly dependent on the detailed morphological appearance and pit pattern in Paris class 0–II colorectal lesions, where early submucosal invasion, lymphovascular invasion and nodal metastatic disease can occur even when the lesion is small [3].

Kato's retrospective review of 4445 patients undergoing magnifying chromoendoscopy examined 3438 lesions classified using the modified Kudo criteria and compared them with either endoscopic or surgically resected specimens [6]. Diagnostic accuracy rates in this series for non-neoplastic lesions, adenomas and invasive carcinomas were 75%, 94% and 85%, respectively [6]. However, despite the large numbers of lesions examined, translation to Western practice was complicated by an adapted Vienna criterion for histopathological classification, which failed to differentiate the grade of dysplastic change in lesions examined [6].

Four prospective studies have addressed the efficacy of magnifying chromoendoscopy in differentiating neoplastic from non-neoplastic colorectal lesions [4, 5, 12]. The study by Tung's group showed a sensitivity and specificity for the differentiation of neoplastic and non-neoplastic lesions of 93.8% and 64.6%, respectively [4]. Furthermore, six neoplastic lesions in this small cohort of 175 were misclassified. In the second prospective analysis, Togashi et al. showed improved sensitivity (92%) and specificity (73%) for the differentiation of neoplastic from non-neoplastic lesions using magnifying chromoendoscopy, with both groups concluding that inadequate operator experience may be responsible for low overall specificity rates [5]. Fu et al. analysed 206 lesions of <10 mm diameter and compared overall diagnostic accuracies with conventional imaging, 0.2% IC, and magnifying chromoendoscopy, using the histological findings as reference. Overall diagnostic accuracy was 84% (173/206) for conventional imaging, 89.3% (184/206) for IC and 95.6% (197/206) for magnifying chromoendoscopy when differentiating neoplastic from non-neoplastic lesions [12]. The largest prospective evaluation of magnifying chromoendoscopy from the Sheffield group prospectively analysed 1008 Paris class 0–II lesions using standardised morphological, pit pattern [3] and histopathological criteria [7]. In this series, the sensitivity and specificity of magnifying chromoendoscopy in distinguishing non-neoplastic from neoplastic lesions was 98% and 92% respectively, but when differentiating neoplastic/non-invasive from neoplastic/invasive lesions sensitivity was poor (50%), with a specificity of 98%.

2.6.2 In Vivo Staging of Colorectal Lesions Using Magnifying Chromoendoscopy

Accurate in vivo staging is essential during colonoscopy (❏ Figs. 2.1–2.4). This approach is particularly important because Paris class 0–II CRCs which are limited to the submucosal layer 1 can be managed by EMR, as the risk of lymphovenous invasion and LNM is <5%. For lesions with deeper vertical invasion, including Paris criteria >1000 μm or stage T2, the risk of LNM increases to 10–15% [13]. EMR in this group is therefore undesirable due to a higher risk of perforation, non-curative excision and untreated nodal disease [2]. Surgical excision is recommended in this group [2].

Chromoscopic colonoscopy used as an in vivo staging tool has been reported by Saitoh et al. [14]. In this retrospective analysis of Paris 0–IIc CRCs, combined videoendoscopy and chromoscopy were used to characterise the essential endoscopic features favoured by lesions invading

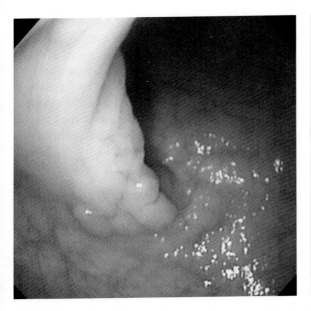

◘ **Fig. 2.1.** Conventional colonoscopic views of the recto-sigmoid junction. There is mucosal nodularity and focal pallor, indicating the possibility of a neoplastic lesion

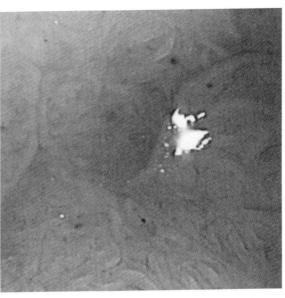

◘ **Fig. 2.3.** High-magnification colonoscopy (100x) shows a neoplastic / non-invasive Kudo type IV crypt pattern. In vivo histopathology would anticipate tubulovillous adenoma with low-moderate grade dysplasia. There is no invasive (type V) crypt architecture to suggest deep submucosal invasion

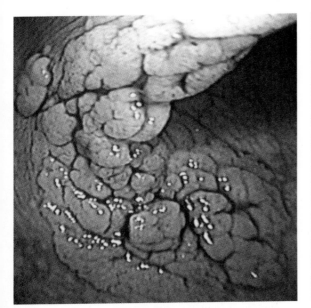

◘ **Fig. 2.2.** Indigo carmine 0.5% chromoscopy clearly delineates the lesion – a lateral spreading tumour Paris class (LST-G)

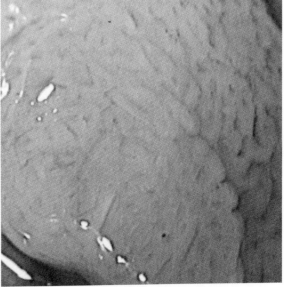

◘ **Fig. 2.4.** High-magnification view of the lesion in retroflexion (100x) shows a non-invasive / neoplastic pattern. A Kudo type IIIL crypt is present. In vivo histopathology would anticipate tubular adenoma with low-grade dysplasia in this segment. The lesion is suitable for endoluminal resection using extended endoscopic mucosal resection or preferably endoscopic submucosal dissection

submucosal layer 1 and 2, which at the time of endoscopy may be used as a tool to guide the colonoscopist's management [14]. Saitoh's criteria include the presence of expansion appearance, depth of surface depression, irregularity and unevenness of the depressed surface and converging folds toward the tumour. Using these criteria, both sensitivity and specificity for determining submucosal layer 2 disease were 90% [14]. However, when 21 lesions showing intramucosal carcinoma were excluded from the analysis, specificity rates fell to 70% [14]. In Hurlstone's prospective analysis of endoscopic morphological anticipation of submucosal invasion in Paris class 0–II lesions [8] using the Nagata subtype [15] analysis of the Kudo type V pit pattern [3], the κ coefficient of agreement between pit type V and histologically confirmed submucosal layer 2 (sm2) invasion was 0.51 (95% CI). Using pit types Vn(B) and Vn(C) as clinical indicators of invasive disease, 97% of lesions were correctly anticipated to have sm2+ invasion; however, specificity was low at 50%, with an overall accuracy of 78% [8]. In the clinical context, such results imply a trend to over-stage lesions, which may deprive some patients of the opportunity of having curative local excision with endoscopic mucosal resection (EMR).

Similar problems have been encountered using the 7.5-MHz ultrasound probe in the staging of rectal carcinoma, with variable accuracy rates reported from 60 to 79%, according to the T-stage system. The introduction of high-frequency 'mini probe' ultrasonography has now been reported to have a high overall accuracy when used to determine submucosal invasion Paris class II lesions. However, ultrasound imaging requires further training, entails significant expense and may prolong the procedure.

2.6.3   Summary of Limitations of Current Technology

- High sensitivity and specificity for the differentiation of non-neoplastic from neoplastic disease but low overall sensitivity for the anticipation of high-grade dysplasia
- Effective over-staging of submucosal layer 3 / T1 neoplasia
- Operator-dependent error
- Surface topographical imaging only
- No ability to image the surface and sub-surface lymphovascular architecture

In these cases, confocal laser endomicroscopy (CLE) might help to overcome the problems. Endomicroscopy enables in vivo histology at subcellular resolution during ongoing endoscopy. Thus, histology is not predicted but can be seen during ongoing endoscopy. Furthermore, in vivo architecture of the mucosal layer can be examined dynamically ranging from the surface to deepest parts of the mucosa. Vessels, connective tissue and epithelial cells can be readily identified and differentiated.

2.7   Chromoscopic Colonoscopy and Magnifying Chromoendoscopy Imaging as an Adjunctive Screening Tool in Colitis

In addition to the detection of sporadic neoplastic lesions of the colorectum, chromoscopic colonoscopy has now been described for the detection of intraepithelial neoplasias (IN) in chronic ulcerative colitis (CUC) (◘ Figs. 2.5 and 2.6). This group is at high risk of CRC with current incidence rates reported between 7 and 30%. CRC complicating CUC accounts for 33% of colitis-related deaths, which forms the rationale for CRC surveillance in patients with longstanding disease [16].

As IN and colitis-associated cancer can occur in macroscopically normal mucosa, random biopsies at 10-cm intervals throughout the colorectum are currently recommended during screening colonoscopy. Historically, the probability for detection of neoplastic change was thought to correlate with the numbers of biopsies taken. However, recent data suggest that pan-chromoscopy using MB can improve the detection of Paris class 0–II and diminutive lesions in CUC when compared with conventional colonoscopic screening protocols alone. Kiesslich et al. showed that chromoscopy permitted a more accurate diagnosis of extent and inflammatory activity in CUC but also enhanced the detection of IN and CRC in colitis ($p=0.0002$ and $p=0.003$, respectively) [17]. Hurlstone et al. have now validated these data using a selective IC chromoscopic technique [18, 19].

Rutter et al. also demonstrated a strong statistical trend towards increased dysplasia detection following IC chromoscopy ($p=0.06$), with a targeted biopsy protocol detecting dysplastic change in significantly more patients than a non-targeted protocol ($p=0.02$) [20]. Furthermore, no dysplasia was detected in 2904 non-targeted biopsies in comparison to a targeted biopsy protocol utilising pan-colonic IC chromoendoscopy [20]. The latter pro-

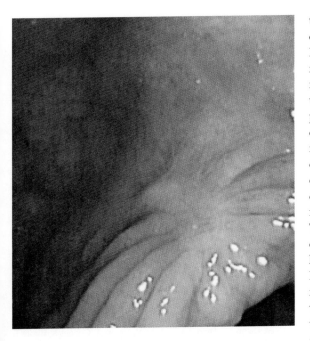

Fig. 2.5. Conventional colonoscopic appearance of the ascending caecal junction in a patient with longstanding chronic ulcerative colitis. There is focal pallor, vascular net loss and striking fold convergence

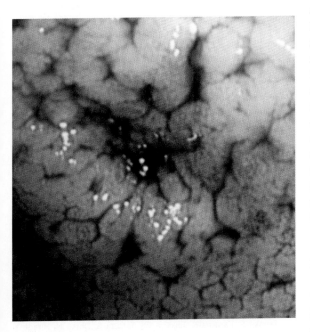

Fig. 2.6. Indigo carmine 0.5% chromoscopy has been applied to the abnormal mucosa that now reveals a Paris 0–II a/c intraepithelial neoplastic lesion. An invasive adenocarcinoma stage pT3/N1 was present on post-surgical histopathology after complete proctocolectomy

tocol required fewer biopsies (157) yet detected nine dysplastic lesions, seven of which were visible only after IC application [20]. The largest prospective data set using magnifying chromoendoscopy and targeted biopsies has recently been published by the Sheffield group [19]. In this series, a total of 350 patients with longstanding pan-colitis (≥8 years duration) underwent surveillance colonoscopy with quadrantic biopsies taken at 10-cm incremental extubation intervals (as per the British Society of Gastroenterology protocol) but with the addition of targeted biopsies of abnormal mucosal areas where defined lesions were further evaluated using a modified Kudo crypt pattern analysis at 100x magnification. These data were then compared with those from 350 disease-duration and disease-extent matched controls who had undergone conventional colonoscopic surveillance. Importantly, more IN lesions were detected in the magnifying chromoendoscopy group than in controls (69 vs. 24, $p<0.0001$). Furthermore, chromoscopy increased the number of Paris class 0–II lesions detected with IN as compared with controls ($p<0.001$). Twenty IN lesions were detected from 12 950 biopsies using conventional colonoscopy (0.15%) with 49/622 (8%) in the magnifying chromoendoscopy targeted group. Of 12 482 biopsies taken in the control group only 18 (0.14%) yielded IN. However, from the targeted biopsy group without magnifying chromoendoscopy imaging, the yield was modestly improved at 1.6% (6/369). Also, using modified Kudo criteria, the sensitivity and specificity were 93% and 88%, respectively, for differentiating neoplastic from non-neoplastic lesions. Total procedure time was significantly longer in the magnification chromoscopic group as compared with controls ($p<0.02$). These data now suggest that chromoscopic colonoscopy is a valid tool for the detection and in vivo classification of IN in CUC and may prompt changes to the current screening guidelines which are labour intensive, time consuming and have a low diagnostic yield.

2.8 Clinical Recommendations and Conclusions

Hence, colonic chromoscopy and magnifying chromoendoscopy are useful tools for discriminating neoplastic and non-neoplastic Paris 0–II colorectal lesions. The decision to target biopsies or progress to therapeutic intervention using EMR can be guided using this technology, and it can avoid inappropriate biopsy or attempted endoscopic resection of lesions without a malignant potential or those which should be referred for surgical excision. Thus, the following endoscopic strategies based upon magnifying chromoendoscopy and pit-pattern analysis can be recommended [11]:

1. Paris class 0–II lesions (<10 mm diameter without a type IIc component and a demonstrable type I/II pit pattern) can be left in situ in the left colon without biopsy.

2. Paris 0–II lesions with a type IIIL/IV pit pattern without an associated type IIc component can be resected in a single-step procedure. This combines histological diagnosis and treatment. A submucosal tattoo can be placed adjacent to the resection site to permit future localisation. A systematic surveillance programme depending on the final histological results should then commence.

3. Lesions with a type IIc component and a type IIIs/V pit pattern either alone or in combination should receive cold biopsy only, even if they are small, and an adjacent mucosal tattoo should be placed for further localisation during surgery or endoscopy. Further evaluation of such lesions using a 20-Mhz ultrasound mini-probe may be helpful in assessing the invasive depth of the lesion, the possibility of LNM, and also may improve safety if elective EMR is an therapeutic option.

In conclusion, the techniques of colonic chromoscopy and magnifying chromoendoscopy have a high overall accuracy for the in vivo histopathological interpretation of sporadic Paris 0–II neoplasia and CUC IN detection, but they are limited to surface topographical imaging only. The techniques are not 100% sensitive or specific, and although they are useful diagnostic tools in vivo, they are not currently a complete replacement for histopathology. It is important for this technology to be developed and used, but requirements for further education and colonoscopic training also need to be addressed. However, in experienced hands, magnifying chromoendoscopy represents a significant advance in colonoscopic practice, which may improve diagnostic yield for significant lesions, lower the burden of insignificant biopsies interpreted by pathologists and enhance therapeutic safety. Confocal laser Endomicroscopy might further refine the characterisation of lesions because it provides in vivo histology [21, 22].

References

1. Paris Workshop Participants (2002) The Paris endoscopic classification of superficial neoplastic lesions: esophagus, stomach and colon. Gastrointest Endosc 58:S3–43
2. Hurlstone DP, Fujii T (2005) Practical uses of chromoendoscopy and magnification at colonoscopy. Gastrointest Endosc Clin N Am 15:687–702
3. Kudo S, Rubio CA, Teixeira CR, Kashida H, Kogure E (2001) Pit pattern in colorectal neoplasia: endoscopic magnifying view. Endoscopy 33:367–373
4. Tung SY, Wu CS, Su MY (2001) Magnifying colonoscopy in differentiating neoplastic from non-neoplastic colorectal lesions. Am J Gastroenterol 96:2628–2632
5. Togashi K, Konishi F, Ishizuka T, Sato T, Senba S, Kanazawa K (1999) Efficacy of magnifying endoscopy in the differential diagnosis of neoplastic and non-neoplastic polyps of the large bowel. Dis Colon Rectum 42:1602–1608
6. Kato S, Fujii T, Koba I, Sano Y, Fu KI, Parra-Blanco A, Tajiri H, Yoshida S, Rembacken B (2001) Assessment of colorectal lesions using magnifying colonoscopy and mucosal dye spraying: can significant lesions be distinguished? Endoscopy 33:306–310
7. Schlemper RJ, Riddell RH, Kato Y, Borchard F, Cooper HS, Dawsey SM, Dixon MF, Fenoglio-Preiser CM, Flejou JF, Geboes K, Hirota T, Itabashi M, Iwafuchi M, Kim YI, Kirchner T, Klimpfinger M, Koike M, Lauwers GY, Lewin KJ, Oberhuber G, Price AB, Rubio CA, Shimoda T, Sipponen P, Stolte M, Watanabe H, Yamabe H (2000) The Vienna classification of gastrointestinal neoplasia. Gut 47:251–255
8. Hurlstone DP, Cross SS, Adam I, Shorthouse AJ, Brown S, Sanders DS, Lobo AJ (2004) Endoscopic morphological anticipation of submucosal invasion in flat and depressed colorectal lesions: clinical implications and subtype analysis of the Kudo type V pit pattern using high-magnification-chromoscopic colonoscopy. Colorectal Dis 6:369–375
9. Kosaka T (1975) Clinico-pathological study of the minute elevated lesion of the colorectal mucosa. J Jpn Soc Coloproctology 8:218–226
10. Nishizawa M (1985) Pertaining to histopathogenesis, growth and progression of early cancer of the colon and rectum in terms of dissecting microscopy and clinical aspects. Stomach Intestine 20:1036–1041
11. Hurlstone DP, Cross SS, Adam I, Shorthouse AJ, Brown S, Sanders DS, Lobo AJ (2004) Efficacy of high magnification chromoscopic colonoscopy for the diagnosis of neoplasia in flat and depressed lesions of the colorectum: a prospective analysis. Gut 53:284–290
12. Fu KI, Sano Y, Kato S, Fujii T, Nagashima F, Yoshino T, Okuno T, Yoshida S, Fujimori T (2004) Chromoendoscopy using indigo carmine dye spraying with magnifying observation is the most reliable method for differential diagnosis between non-neoplastic and neoplastic colorectal lesions: a prospective study. Endoscopy 36:1089–1093
13. Tanaka S, Haruma K, Teixeira CR, Tatsuta S, Ohtsu N, Hiraga Y, Yoshihara M, Sumii K, Kajiyama G, Shimamoto F (1995) Endoscopic treatment of submucosal invasive colorectal carcinoma with special reference to risk factors for lymph node metastasis. J Gastroenterol 30:710–717

14. Saitoh Y, Obara T, Watari J, Nomura M, Taruishi M, Orii Y, Taniguchi M, Ayabe T, Ashida T, Kohgo Y (1998) Invasion depth diagnosis of depressed type early colorectal cancers by combined use of videoendoscopy and chromoendoscopy. Gastrointest Endosc 48:362–370

15. Nagata S, Tanaka S, Haruma K, Yoshihara M, Sumii K, Kajiyama G, Shimamoto F (2000) Pit pattern diagnosis of early colorectal carcinoma by magnifying colonoscopy: clinical and histological implications. Int J Oncol 16:927–934

16. Eaden JA, Abrams KR, Mayberry JF (2001) The risk of colorectal cancer in ulcerative colitis: a meta-analysis. Gut 48:526–535

17. Kiesslich R, Fritsch J, Holtmann M, Koehler HH, Stolte M, Kanzler S, Nafe B, Jung M, Galle PR, Neurath MF (2003) Methylene blue-aided chromoendoscopy for the detection of intraepithelial neoplasia and colon cancer in ulcerative colitis. Gastroenterology 124:880–888

18. Hurlstone DP, Cross SS (2005) Role of aberrant crypt foci detected using high-magnification chromoscopic colonoscopy in human colorectal carcinogenesis. J Gastroenterol Hepatol 20 (2):173-181

19. Hurlstone DP, Sanders DS, Lobo AJ, McAlindon ME, Cross SS (2005) Indigo carmine-assisted high-magnification chromoscopic colonoscopy for the detection and characterisation of intraepithelial neoplasia in ulcerative colitis: a prospective evaluation. Endoscopy 37:1186–1192

20. Rutter MD, Saunders BP, Schofield G, Forbes A, Price AB, Talbot IC (2004) Pancolonic indigo carmine dye spraying for the detection of dysplasia in ulcerative colitis. Gut 53:256–260

21. Hurlstone DP, Thomson M, Brown S, Tiffin N, Cross SS, Hunter MD. Confocal Endomicroscopy in Ulcerative Colitis: Differentiating Dysplasia-Associated Lesional Mass and Adenoma-Like Mass. Clin Gastroenterol Hepatol. 2007 Aug 7; [Epub ahead of print]

22. Hurlstone DP, Kiesslich R., Thomson, Atkinson R, Cross SS. Confocal chromoscopic endomicroscopy is superior to chromoscopy alone for the detection and characterisation of intraepithelial neoplasia in chronic ulcerative colitis: a randomised controlled study. Gut 2007 (in press)

Development and Current Technological Status of Confocal Laser Endomicroscopy

Peter Delaney, Steven Thomas, Wendy McLaren

Key concepts:

- Fibre-optic confocal microscopy is utilising a single optical fibre as both the illumination and detection confocal pinholes.
- This concept is currently used in confocal laser endomicroscopy.
- Endomicroscopy combines confocal microscopy with conventional endoscopy to provide real-time interactivity between simultaneous macroscopic and microscopic imaging.
- Endomicroscopy provides volumetric sampling - the »virtual biopsy«

3.1 Introduction

This chapter aims to explain the principles of confocal microscopy, the reasons for the key features in the present form of endomicroscopy, and how they account for what is seen during practical endomicroscopy of the GI tract.

After reading this chapter, the reader should understand:

- The basic concepts of confocal microscopy
- Key developments that have enabled and shaped the transition from bench-top microscopy to clinical endomicroscopy as we know it today
- The current implementation of the technology used to generate the images documented throughout this atlas
- How endomicroscopy visualises the three-dimensional microarchitectural features of the various GI mucosae
- Volumetric imaging and the concept of the »virtual biopsy«

Marvin Minsky invented confocal microscopy in the late 1950s [1]; however, it is only in recent years that the refinement and miniaturisation required to allow practical real-time microscopy during ongoing endoscopy was achieved.

Minsky, a neuroscientist, wished to document the three-dimensional architecture and interconnections of neurons in thick pieces of brain. This was not possible with microscopes of the day, due to the depth of field limitations and out-of-focus blur artefacts encountered in high-magnification optics. He proposed the use of spatial filters (pinholes) and scanning to dissect and isolate the focal plane of an optical microscope, which would thus allow clear imaging of focal plane information within thick tissue specimens, even living tissue in vivo.

Although his concepts were sound and underpin even modern confocal microscopes, technical limitations prevented viable implementations of the idea at that time. In the absence of fast electromechanical scanning actuators, lasers, high-sensitivity detectors and digital image acquisition, the technique was impractical.

It was some three decades later (after such technologies had become commonplace) that point scanning laser confocal microscope systems were developed and became commercially available. The ability to »optically section« a piece of intact tissue without physically disrupting it is immensely powerful for observing the micromachinations of life. It is thus not surprising that such instruments rapidly became important and popular tools in cell biology.

With widespread availability of bench-top confocal microscopes, the possibilities for non-destructive microscopy as a form of medical examination also became obvious. However, conventional confocal microscopes were large, bulky instruments designed for the laboratory researcher, precluding most conceivable applications in medical examination, especially those requiring endoscopic access to internal organs. Further breakthroughs in miniaturisation were made (mostly throughout the 1990s), and these enabled the 'reinvention' of confocal microscopy as a medical imaging modality.

Every stage of technical development has been driven by the realities of imaging living tissues in vivo, as encountered through both animal and early human studies, including imaging of the human skin, the uterine cervix, front of the eye and the oral cavity, abdominal organs accessed during laparoscopic and open surgery and, of course, the GI mucosa. This has also resulted in development of key protocols for the use of clinical fluorescent contrast agents and instrumentation features and workflows not found in desktop confocal microscopes but essential for clinical endomicroscopy.

Thus, although sharing common founding principles, clinical endomicroscopes bear little resemblance to their desktop ancestors. The following sections outline both the foundation principles of confocal microscopy and the particular technological approach and features that have enabled the field of practical GI endomicroscopy as documented in this atlas.

3.2 Principles of Confocal Microscopy

A common characteristic of magnifying optics is that the depth of field is reduced with increasing magnification and resolution. Anyone who has attempted macrophotography of very small objects will appreciate the inability to focus on foreground and background objects at the same time. When a small insect on a flower is imaged, for example, the underlying plant life is out of focus.

At microscopic magnification, this is even more pronounced, and the depth of field is reduced to microns. If a classical microscope is used to examine intact, translucent, living tissue, any structure in the focal plane is swamped by blur and flare from the overlying or underlying out-of-focus tissue.

In practice, this requires tissue to be cut into thin sections comparable in thickness to the depth of field (or focal plane thickness) of the microscope and mounted onto glass slides for examination. This is, of course, common practice for examination of biopsy tissue in the histopathology laboratory.

Point scanning confocal microscopes obviate this requirement by the use of a particular geometrical optical configuration and scanning that dissects and isolates the focal plane of the microscope, one point at a time.

◘ Figure 3.1 diagrams the optical principle that achieves this focal plane isolation. A light source (typically a laser) is configured as a point source that is focused by a microscope objective lens to a diffraction limited spot in the tissue. Light that is scattered, or fluorescence excited and emitted, at the focus in the sample will partially return back through the optics along the path from which it arrived (if left undeviated, it would focus back to the point source by reciprocity). A beam-splitter placed into the path reflects the return light towards a detector. The optics will focus the light from the focal point in the specimen to its conjugate focus near the detector. A pinhole is placed at this point, allowing the light from the focal point to pass through to the detector and be measured. However, light from anywhere else in the specimen will not be projected to this same point and will be rejected by the aperture. The point source of light, the detection pinhole, and the focal point in the specimen are all conjugate foci, hence the term confocal.

A scanning system introduced into the forward/reverse optical path moves the spot around in the sample. This is typically performed in a raster pattern under con-

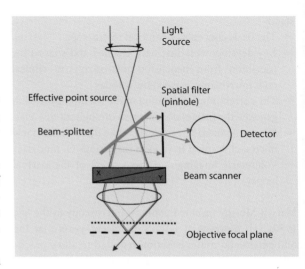

◘ **Fig. 3.1.** Basic principle of confocal microscopy

trol of a computer system that synchronously digitises the detector signal for reconstruction into an image.

Importantly, the resultant image contains signal only from the focal plane and is free of out-of-focus blur and flare. In a confocal microscope image, objects do not »go out of focus«, but rather disappear or become black. This ability to isolate the focal plane is termed »optical sectioning«, and is the key feature that empowers this form of microscopy over conventional magnifying optics for the examination of intact, translucent tissue.

Of course, the focal plane is not required to be at the surface of the tissue – any plane within the tissue (within limits of light propagation posed by absorption and scattering) will be isolated from overlying or underlying structures.

Furthermore, if this plane is moved to different depths in the tissue, images from sequential planes can be collected, and such an image set represents a three-dimensional volume in the tissue. This is an important capability for endoscopy and will be explained further below.

3.3 Miniaturisation – Fibre-Optic Confocal Microscopy

Confocal microscopy applications such as imaging of the endoscopically accessed GI tract require extreme miniaturisation of the microscope imaging head. This has required the combination of several enabling technologies and numerous practical refinements, including the use of specialised optical fibres as confocal pinholes and the development of miniature scanners, image depth actuators, dedicated objective lenses and a uniquely integrated endoscope with both macroscopic and microscopic imaging capabilities.

Delaney et al. [2, 3] developed fibre-optic confocal microscopy utilising a single optical fibre functioning as both the illumination and detection confocal pinholes (as used in the present endomicroscopy system diagrammed in ☐ Fig. 3.2). Laser light is projected into the fibre, which in turn projects the light through a focusing lens into the tissue. Light returning from the focus can be efficiently recaptured into the same fibre for transmission back to the

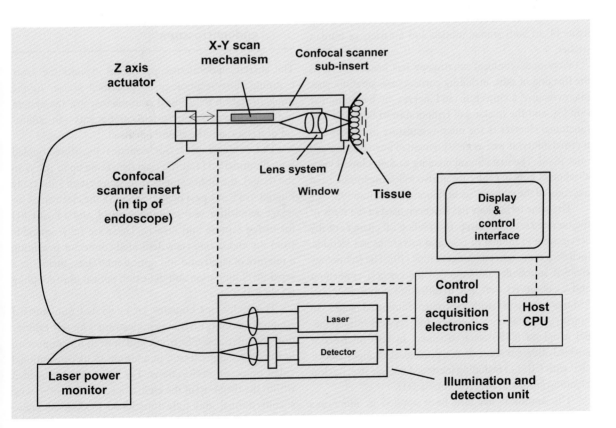

☐ **Fig. 3.2.** System diagram for current generation of scanning fibre endomicroscope

proximal end, where it is then separated onto a detector. Light emanating from regions of tissue outside the focused spot does not focus back into the fibre and is thus largely rejected from detection. The fibre output is then scanned point-wise as a computer synchronously digitises the detector signal to build up the confocal image (◻ Fig. 3.2).

As the illumination and detection apertures are the same physical entity, and the separation of the forward and return light paths is not part of the scan mechanism, this approach facilitates miniaturisation of the scanning unit and eliminates numerous optical alignments required in bulk optical confocal microscopes. This approach was pioneered by Optiscan Imaging in Australia, who have developed several generations of progressively miniaturised fibre-optic confocal microscopes based on this technology, enabling bench-top confocal microscopes, handheld scanners for dermatological imaging, rigid confocal colposcopes and arthroscopes, and most recently a scanner small enough to allow integration into a flexible gastrointestinal endoscope.

The miniaturisation offered by the fibre-optic approach has become well established for the examination of living tissue [4] in both animal models and a variety of human studies.

Fibre-optic confocal microscopy has been applied to the imaging of skin, including corneocytes, keratinocytes, microvascular architecture and nerves in living mouse skin [5], and the tracking of temporal morphological and functional changes in the microvasculature in response to thermal injury, as well as measurement of burn thickness in mice [6–8]. The first clinical imaging studies allowed visualisation of human epidermis in vivo following intradermal injection of the contrast agent fluorescein sodium [9].

The same technology has also been used in the study of the uterine cervix. In sheep, morphological changes of the cervix were examined in response to various sex steroids, including oestrogen and progesterone [10]. The technology enabled subcellular resolution of the cervical epithelium and lay observers were able to differentiate morphological features associated with oestrogen-dominated states. In human subjects, normal cervix and cervical intraepithelial neoplasia (CIN) were visualised. In vivo microscopy enabled differentiation of morphological changes associated with CIN1–3 including increased nuclear size, nuclear pleomorphism and hyperchromasia [11].

The approach has also been applied in numerous animal studies in the colon. Delaney et al. first assessed the suitability of using confocal imaging for subsurface structures within the colon, both in vitro using human and rat biopsies and in vivo in rats [12, 13]. Papworth et al. [14] used fibre-optic confocal microscopy to visualise the subsurface morphology of nerves and blood vessels in the rat colon in vivo. The nerve ganglia, primary fibre tracts and neuronal cell bodies were all examined using confocal microscopy.

In vivo microscopy in a rat ulcerative colitis model documented cellular mucosal changes [15] and microvascular changes [16] associated with early disease progression. These studies demonstrated the key surface and subsurface cellular changes that are directly observable with endomicroscopy in the three-dimensional volume of tissue at and near the surface of the colonic mucosa. These data also documented, for the first time, the use of a simple image classification system enabling blinded observers to accurately grade pathology from confocal images obtained in vivo. These data served as key inputs to the imaging parameters ultimately developed for human GI endomicroscopy.

3.4 Current Technology in the flexible GI endomicroscope

The current endomicroscopy system exploits the same scanning fibre technology as described above. In the implementation for clinical endomicroscopy, the system is divided into two main system components – the confocal processor and the endoscope itself.

The confocal processor contains the fibre-coupled laser illumination (488-nm laser delivering up to 1 mW to the tissue), the fibre-coupled detection system (spectrally filtered to a band-pass of 505–585 nm), the electronics for image acquisition and scanning control, and a host CPU for image capture and display. These are fully separable from the endoscope via a dedicated connector providing a mixture of electronic and optical interfaces, including a separate illumination and detection optical fibre coupling (◻ Fig. 3.2).

The endoscope contains an integrated miniaturised confocal scanning mechanism, electronics for self-calibration and interfaces (electronic and optical) for connection to the confocal processor, in addition to its conventional video processor connections. The scanner is embedded within the distal tip of the endoscope, which is otherwise a conventional and fully functioned flexible GI endoscope, the operational details of which will be covered in the next chapter.

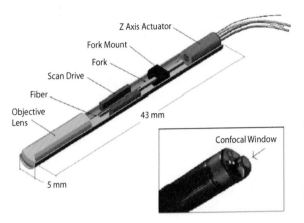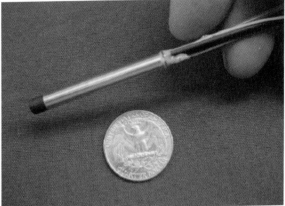

□ **Fig. 3.3.** Miniature fibre-optic confocal x,y,z scanner for flexible endoscopy, shown diagrammatically (*left*), as a complete device (*right*) and packaged into a Pentax flexible endomicroscope (*inset, left*)

In the scanner, the optical fibre is mounted on an electromagnetically driven resonant tuning fork, which scans the fibre in the x (horizontal) axis. The fork is also part of a cantilever, which provides y (vertical) axis movement of the fibre tip. This combination produces a raster scan of the fibre. A custom-designed miniature objective lens projects the illumination and return light between the fibre and tissue. These components are all mounted into a single inner assembly of the scanner.

The z (image depth) axis is controlled by a compact actuator based on shape memory alloy technology, and moves the diagrammed components within a windowed outer sleeve over a depth range of approximately 250 μm. This is configured such that the outer window can be placed into stationary contact with the surface of the mucosa, and the imaging depth mechanism moves the inner assembly to project the imaging plane to different depths within the tissue. The inner scanner components, overall scanner assembly and integration into the tip of an endoscope are shown in □ Fig. 3.3.

3.5 Current Technology – Key Features for Endomicroscopy of the GI Tract

The confocal images produced by the scanner are orientated en face to the tissue surface. The physical contact between the tip of the scanner and the mucosa provides alignment of the scanned image to the tissue surface in most situations, as well as creating stability for microscopic imaging.

Endomicroscopy images contain high information content. The scanner provides up to 1024 x 1024-pixel (1 megapixel) confocal images, representing a lateral field of view of approximately 500 μm x 500 μm with 0.7 μm lateral resolution. This field of view is large enough to appreciate tissue architectural patterns such as crypt patterns (for example, 9–16 colonic crypts are visible within a single image of colonic mucosa), yet detailed enough to offer true cellular, subcellular, and in some cases even subnuclear detail within those patterns.

This is extremely important, since the broader architectural features visible by close examination with the conventional endoscope also appear in the microscopic images as a framework within which the cellular detail can be interpreted. By way of example, pit patterns observed macroscopically will be clearly visible in the microscopic images, but replete with cellular details such as epithelial cell stratification, basement membrane alignment/integrity, and microvascular details such as uniformity of capillary diameters.

The axial resolution (»optical section thickness«) is approximately 7 μm in the current scanner. In most GI mucosae, this relates to around one to two cell layers per image. This thickness ideally allows visualisation of congruent layers of cellular structure and planar microvascular networks. In fact, the en face alignment achieved by contact with the tissue allows routine visualisation of patent microvasculature in a form that is not possible in conventional histology of biopsies.

Scanning occurs at interactive speed with progressive lines displayed as they are scanned, with a trade-off between speed and resolution. Scan rates range from several frames per second for sub-megapixel resolutions to 0.8 frames/s for full 1 megapixel resolution. This enables real-time interaction with the image and rapid sampling of the tissue.

The focal plane depth relative to the contact surface can be dynamically adjusted while one is imaging from the surface to deeper layers, down to a maximum depth of 250 µm deep with control to around 4-µm increments. Although it is technically feasible to scan comprehensive three-dimensional volumes in this fashion, typically collection of three to four key depths containing certain features of importance provides a rapid representation of a small volume of tissue.

As this sampling truly captures information from both surface and subsurface regions of a small volume of tissue, it can be regarded as a »virtual biopsy«, taking several seconds to collect, depending on the number of depths sampled.

This »virtual biopsy« concept is fundamentally important. The features of the instrument combine to provide a field of view, interactive scanning, control of depth and digital image collection that enable rapid sampling of the tissue with sampling statistics that are superior to those associated with the collection of conventional biopsies.

Depth of imaging achievable by confocal microscopy is very dependent on both the tissue and the contrast agent protocol employed.

Formation of a confocal image depends upon projection of a tightly focused beam of laser light into the tissue, as well as on recovery and projection of emitted light back toward the confocal detection aperture (the optical fibre in this case). This optical path is susceptible to the light propagation, absorption and scattering properties of the tissue. As such, it is impossible to predict an exact limit of optical penetration. Scattering will also decrease the image resolution and sensitivity with increasing depth in the tissue.

These effects are observed as a progressive softening and darkening of the image as the imaging plane depth approaches its practical limit while it is moved through the upper 100–200 µm of tissue.

As a fluorescence imaging modality, the confocal image is not so much a direct representation of the cel-lular structures themselves, but rather the distribution of fluorescent chemicals relative to those cells and their matrix. Such fluorescence may be endogenous or exogenous; however, the vast majority of clinical endomicroscopy data to date relate to the use of exogenous fluorescent contrast agents.

3.6   Summary and »Take-home« messages

The refinement of the technology for GI endoscopy is impressive and has resulted in excellent clinical results, as reported elsewhere in this volume.

Such studies have enabled clear true in vivo histology in over ten indications at the time of ongoing endoscopy. There is a strong relationship between the technical performance of this modality and the essential histological elements that are observable in the major mucosae of the GI tract. These fundamental issues are important for appreciating the incredible diversity of histological data obtainable in multiple pathologies.

The key take-home messages can thus be summarised as follows:

- Endomicroscopy and desk-top confocal microscopy share the same principles but are implemented for completely different workflows.
- The endomicroscope has been developed for rapid sampling of both cellular detail and tissue architecture.
- Surface and subsurface imaging provides volumetric sampling – the »virtual biopsy«.
- Endomicroscopy is a fluorescence modality whereby different contrast agents can elucidate different details.
- Endomicroscopy combines confocal microscopy with conventional endoscopy to provide real-time interactivity between simultaneous macroscopic and microscopic imaging.

References

1. Minsky M (1957) US Patent # 3013467, Microscopy Apparatus
2. Delaney PM, Harris, MR, King, RG (1994) Fiber-optic laser scanning confocal microscope suitable for fluorescence imaging. Appl Optics 33:573–577
3. Delaney PM, Harris MR (1995) Fiberoptics in confocal microscopy. In: Pawley JB (ed) Handbook of biological confocal microscopy. Plenum, New York, pp 515–523

4. Delaney PM, Papworth GD, King RG (1998) Fibre optic confocal imaging (FOCI) for in vivo subsurface microscopy of the colon. In: Preedy VR, Watson RR (eds) Methods in disease: investigating the gastrointestinal tract. Greenwich Medical Media Ltd (London, distributed by Oxford University Press) Chap. 15, pp 169–178

5. Bussau LJ, Vo LT, Delaney PM, Papworth GD, Barkla DH, King RG (1998) Fibre optic confocal imaging (FOCI) of keratinocytes, blood vessels and nerves in hairless mouse skin in vivo. J Anat 192:187–194

6. Vo LT, Papworth GD, Delaney PM, Barkla DH, King RG (1998) A study of vascular response on thermal injury on hairless mice by fibre optic confocal imaging, laser Doppler flowmetry and conventional histology. Burns 24:319–324

7. Vo LT, Papworth GD, Delaney PM, Barkla DH, King RG (2000) In vivo mapping of the vascular changes in skin burns of anaesthetised mice by fibre optic confocal imaging (FOCI). J Dermatol Sci 23:46–52

8. Vo LT, Anikijenko P, McLaren WJ, Delaney PM, Barkla DH, King RG (2001) Autofluorescence of skin burns detected by fiber-optic confocal imaging: evidence that cool water treatment limits progressive thermal damage in anaesthetised hairless mice. J Trauma 51:98–104

9. Swindle LD, Thomas SG, Freeman M, Delaney PM (2003) View of normal human skin in vivo as observed using fluorescent fibre-optic confocal microscopic imaging. J Invest Dermatol 121 (4):706-712

10. Bott EM, Young IR, Jenkin G, McLaren WJ (2006) Detection of morphological changes of the ovine cervix in response to sex steroids using a fluorescence confocal endomicroscope. Am J Obstet Gynecol 194:105–112

11. McLaren WJ, Tan J, Quinn M (2003) Detection of cervical neoplasia using non-invasive fibre-optic confocal microscopy. 5th International Multidisciplinary Congress – Eurogin (Paris, France), Article D413C0014, pp 213–217

12. Delaney PM, Harris MR, King RG (1993) Novel microscopy using fibre optic confocal imaging and its suitability for subsurface blood vessel imaging in vivo. Clin Exp Pharmacol Physiol 20:197–198

13. Delaney PM, King RG, Lambert JR, Harris MR (1994) Fibre optic confocal imaging (FOCI) for subsurface microscopy of the colon in vivo. J Anat 184:157–160

14. Papworth GD, Delaney PM, Bussau LJ, Vo LT, King RG (1998) In vivo fibre optic confocal imaging of microvasculature and nerves in the rat vas deferens and colon. J Anat 192:489–495

15. McLaren WJ, Anikijenko P, Barkla D, Delaney PM, King RG (2001) In vivo detection of experimental ulcerative colitis in rats using fiberoptic confocal imaging (FOCI). Dig Dis Sci 46:263–2276

16. McLaren WJ, Anikijenko P, Thomas SG, Delaney PM, King RG (2002) In vivo detection of morphological and microvascular changes of the colon in association with colitis using fiberoptic confocal imaging (FOCI). Dig Dis Sci 47:2424–2433

Examination Technique of Confocal Laser Endomicroscopy

Martin Goetz, Kerry Dunbar, Marcia I. Canto

Key concepts:
- The confocal endomicroscope has two unique buttons: button 3 to reset to home position and button 4 for control of scanning.
- The resolution of endomicroscopic images is up to 1024 × 1024 pixels.
- Fluorescein and/or acriflavine are used as fluorescent agents for endomicroscopy.

4.1 Introduction

The first publication about a confocal fluorescence microscope integrated into the distal tip of a conventional colonoscope (Pentax EC 3830FK, Tokyo, Japan) appeared in 2004 [1], showing that in vivo microscopy at subcellular resolution (0.7 μm) simultaneously displayed with white-light endoscopy had become possible. Today, endomicroscopy can be performed in the upper and lower GI tract [2–10]. This chapter deals with the examination technique of confocal laser endomicroscopy.

4.2 The Confocal Endomicroscope

Confocal laser endomicroscopy (CLE) is possible due to a miniaturised laser scanning microscope which has been integrated into the distal tip of an otherwise conventional video endoscope (for specifications, ◘ Table 4.1).

The buttons of the hand piece on the front function like standard endoscope buttons for freeze and image capture. On the back of the control head are two additional control buttons (buttons 3 and 4) that are unique to the endomicroscope. The location of the control knobs 3 and

4 is shown in ◘ Fig. 4.1. One click of the button on the back-left (button 4) causes the confocal imaging direction to return to the Home position approximately 10 μm deep

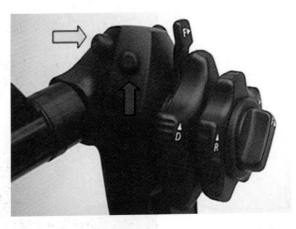

◘ **Fig. 4.1.** Controls unique to the confocal endomicroscope. The locations of the control knobs 3 (*right*) and 4 (*left*) are indicated by two *arrows*. These buttons are unique to confocal laser endomicroscopy and control the scanning depth. One click of the button on the back-left (button 4) causes the confocal imaging direction to return to the »home position« approximately 10 μm deep from the surface

4

▣ **Table 4.1.** Specifications of the confocal laser endoscope	
Tip diameter	12.8 mm
Tip angulation	Up/down 130 degrees, left/right 120 degrees
Insertion tube diameter	12.8 mm
Working length	1300, 1500, 1700 mm
Control body knobs	
Front-top, button 1	Freeze
Front-bottom, button 2	Picture
Back-right, button 3 (red arrow, Fig. 1a)	1 click – reset to home position 2 clicks – put processor on standby (prior to use of electrocautery)
Back-left, button 4 (yellow arrow, Fig. 1a)	1 click – move scanning plane 1 section deep from the surface 2 clicks – reverse scanning direction

from the surface. This is a useful function if you get »lost« and are unsure about whether you are in the superficial or deep mucosa. Button 3 is used all the time during endomicroscopic imaging to move the scanning direction one plane up or down, depending upon the direction of imaging.

A confocal imaging window at the distal tip of the endoscope provides the function of a cover slip (▣ Fig. 4.2). Note that the confocal imaging window is located 5 mm to the left of the biopsy channel. This is important for targeting biopsy after endomicroscopic imaging.

The outer diameter of the endoscope is 12.8 mm, that of the working channel is 2.8 mm. The endoscope contains a conventional charge-coupled device (CCD) chip for macroscopic white-light imaging. The endoscopy system tower consists of two monitors for simultaneous display of videoendoscopic and endomicroscopic images (▣ Fig. 4.3). Apart from the usual white-light system requirements, the confocal system has an additional

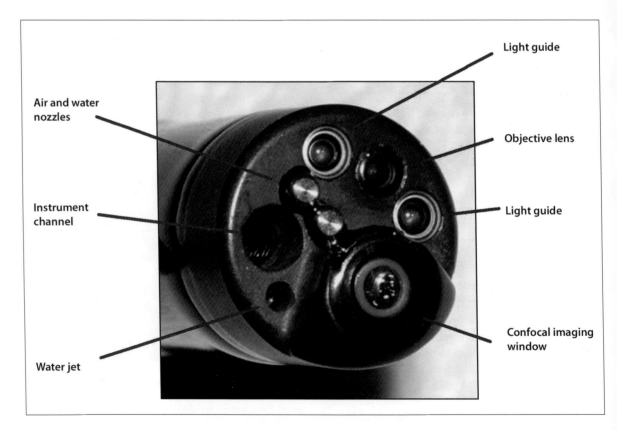

▣ **Fig. 4.2.** The distal tip of the confocal endomicroscope contains the scan mechanism and the confocal imaging window. The instrument channel measures 2.8 mm, the outer diameter of the endoscope is 13.2 mm. The endomicrosope contains two light guides

optical unit and computer unit, to which the laser and detector lines are connected via plugs.

A solid-state laser provides an excitation wavelength of 488 nm that is focused onto a distinct imaging plane within the tissue. Infiltration depth of the blue laser light is 0–250 μm, and the optical slice thickness is 7 μm, with lateral and axial resolution of 0.7 μm. The laser power output at the tissue surface can be adapted to the tissue contrast from 0 to 1000 μW. The microscopic field of view is 475 x 475 μm. Images are captured at a frame rate of 1.6 images/s at a resolution of 1024 x 512 pixels, or at 0.8 images/s at a resolution of 1024 x 1024 pixels.

Cleaning the confocal endomicroscope is similar to cleaning conventional endoscopes. The tip of the endoscope contains the scanning head and should be handled with special care to avoid trauma that might damage the endomicroscope by offsetting the scan mechanism or z-axis actuator. For protection of the confocal endoscope, a soft cap is provided for cleaning in automated

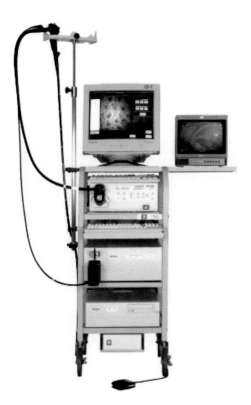

□ Fig. 4.3. Videoendoscopic and endomicroscopic images are displayed simultaneously. Confocal images are captured with the help of a foot pedal

endoscope washing machines. The laser and computer unit plugs are secured with metal caps. No additional safety or hygiene regulations are required for the confocal endoscope.

4.3   Patient Preparation

For confocal endomicroscopy of the upper and lower GI tract, patients are prepared as for routine endoscopy. No additional mucolytic agent is needed for endomicroscopic visualisation of the upper GI tract. If necessary, the mucosa can be cleared of mucus by a water jet, and gastric juice can be removed by suctioning to obtain a good contact of the endomicroscope with the mucosa. For the lower GI tract, the bowel cleansing by ingestion of an oral electrolyte lavage solution required for normal colonoscopy is sufficient preparation for confocal endomicroscopy. However, excellent bowel preparation is mandatory, as stool remnants might have inherent autofluorescence and interfere with detection of tissue fluorescence. In addition, similar to videoendoscopic imaging, poor bowel preparation necessitates more frequent cleaning of the confocal imaging window and disturbs the detection of the suspicious lesions that are to be investigated by confocal endomicroscopy.

Panendomicroscopy of the colon is not feasible, considering that the endomicroscopic field of view is 475 x 475 μm. Therefore, endomicroscopy in a clinical setting always consists of the combination of white-light endoscopy (macroscopy) and confocal laser endomicroscopy (microscopy). In addition, endomicroscopy can be combined with a contrast-enhancing method for identification and targeting of suspicious lesions in situations where a large area of the intestine is to be monitored (e.g. in colonoscopy for ulcerative colitis cancer surveillance). Chromoendoscopy with methylene blue or indigo carmine has been successfully combined with confocal imaging of the lower GI tract [1]. While the uptake of methylene blue into the cytoplasm of epithelial cells can be visualised and indigo carmine is applied as a contrast agent of chromoendoscopy, these do not interfere with confocal imaging.

However, contrast enhancement with acetic acid, which is frequently used for evaluation of Barrett's oesophagus, causes intermittent changes in the epithelial surface structure which blurs confocal images and cannot be recommended for confocal imaging Since imaging using fluorescein is pH-dependent (see below), acetic acid contrast enhancement further impedes confocal imaging.

4.4   In Vivo Confocal Imaging

Macroscopic videoendoscopic imaging with the confocal endomicroscope is identical to conventional videoendoscopy, and handling of the confocal endoscope corresponds to that of a conventional colonoscope or gastroscope. However, flexion of the distal end is restricted owing to the longer rigid part.

The confocal imaging window is slightly prominent at the distal tip of the endoscope and can therefore be visualised in the videoendoscopic image at the left lower corner (◘ Fig. 4.4). This is used to macroscopically target lesions under videoendoscopic control. The endomicroscope within the distal tip of the endoscope produces a black protrusion on the video screen, which beginning confocal endoscopists may sometimes mistake for the lumen of the non-inflated colon. From this confocal imaging window, a blue laser light beam can be seen in the videoendoscopic image, scanning the mucosal surface (◘ Fig. 4.4). Videoendoscopic and endomicroscopic images are displayed simultaneously on two separate screens. Confocal images can be captured with the help of a foot pedal and are digitally stored (◘ Fig. 4.3).

Compared with a conventional videoendoscope, the tip of the endomicroscopy scope is slightly less flexible since the miniaturised laser scanner has been integrated into the distal 4 cm of the colonoscope. This might require some practice in advancing the scope through sharper sigmoid bends, but caecal intubation is usually easily achieved. Almost full-scale inversion (130°) is possible for retroflexion in the rectum or to visualise the upper portion of the stomach by turning both wheels in opposite directions. However, due to the limitation of angulation, some parts of the fundus and cardia are difficult or sometimes impossible to investigate [4]. Intubation of the terminal ileum is achieved at rates similar to those with conventional colonoscopy [6].

For endomicroscopic imaging, the confocal imaging window is placed directly onto the area of interest. The highest imaging quality is obtained by achieving full vertical contact of the confocal imaging window with the mucosa through angulation of the tip of the endoscope. Movement artefacts are the main source of reduced confocal image quality, so a stable interface between the tissue

and the confocal imaging window is absolutely necessary (◘ Fig. 4.5). Intermittent suppression of peristalsis by N-butyl-scopolamine or glucagon can be helpful in obtaining stable contact, but imaging can still be challenging in some patients at the gastro-oesophageal junction due to respiratory and cardiac motion. Stable positioning of the confocal imaging window relative to the area of interest can usually be achieved by a slight angulation (about 45°) and subsequent mild pressure of the tip of the endoscope onto the mucosa. Applying continuous suction helps to further stabilise the confocal image. By using the wheels of the endoscope, the tip can be carefully moved across the lesion to image all fields of a suspicious area. By using the z-axis actuator, the scanning depth of the laser light can be regulated, which results in complete three-dimensional microscopic resolution of a lesion or the mucosal layer. When suction is applied, the post-suction intramucosal haemorrhage or polyp is located 5 mm from the area that has been examined by confocal endomicroscopy. Therefore, if a biopsy is warranted for ex vivo correlation, it should be taken exactly 5 mm to the left of the suction polyp.

While conventional ex vivo histology of biopsy specimens are usually oriented to yield a transverse, perpendicular section through the mucosa, the endomicroscopist evaluates en face optical tissue sections that run parallel to the tissue surface (◘ Fig. 4.6). The examiner should aim to obtain an immediate diagnosis from the

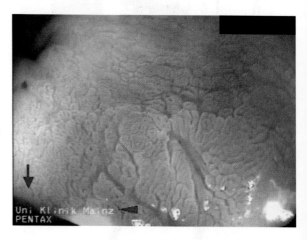

◘ **Fig. 4.4.** The confocal imaging window protudes from the seven o'clock position at the distal tip of the endoscope (*arrow*). This is used to target lesions under videoendoscopic control. When the confocal imaging window is not put onto the mucosa, a blue laser light can be identified emanating from the laser scanner (*arrowhead*). The example shows examination of non-neoplastic Barrett's oesophagus.

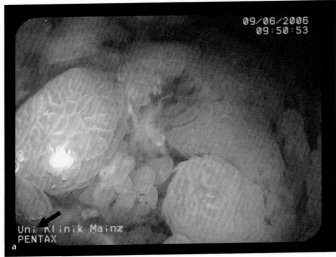

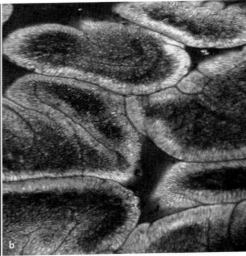

Fig. 4.5a,b. Positioning of the confocal microscope. **a** The confocal microscope is visible at the left lower corner of the white-light endoscopic image (*arrow*). The area of interest has to be targeted with the endomicroscope. **b** Confocal images represent the tissue touched with the microscope. Sometimes continuous suction is mandatory to achieve full contact with tissue over the whole confocal microscopic window. A stable position is mandatory if an optical biopsy (confocal images from the surface and deeper parts of the tissue) is to be obtained

Conventional histology: Transverse section

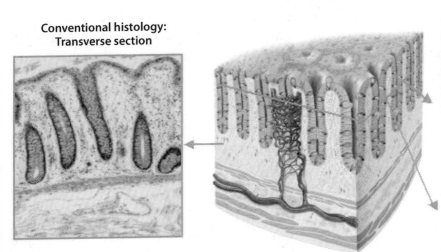

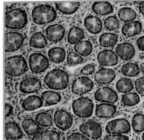

In vivo confocal microscopy: en face fiew

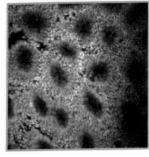

Fig. 4.6. In conventional histopathology, the specimen is cut into thin transverse slices, yielding a transverse section through the biopsies (*left*: H & E stain of normal colonic mucosa). Confocal endomicroscopy results in an optical section that runs parallel to the tissue surface, corresponding to an en face view onto the mucosa (*right, upper panel*: H & E stain of normal colonic mucosa, *lower panel*: topcial acriflavine). (*Schematic diagram* courtesy of Optiscan Pty, Ltd, Australia)

generated images to take advantage of in vivo histology during the ongoing examination. Interpretation of the confocal images requires a thorough knowledge of the normal and abnormal microscopic architecture of the upper and lower gastrointestinal tract; with pattern recognition rather than a minute appreciation of every subtle cellular detail common for early interpretation of normal and abnormal confocal imaging. To this end, confocal pattern classification systems have been established for the upper and lower gastrointestinal tract. They are based on the evaluation of the microvascular and crypt or glandular architecture, which are described in detail in the following chapters. The classification systems are easy to learn, easy to apply, allow an accurate and fast tissue diagnosis, and show good inter- and intra-observer agreement. Imaging depth of the currently used instruments is limited to 250 μm. Therefore, only the mucosa can be scanned while the submucosal layer cannot regularly be visualised. While learning confocal endomicroscopy (cf. ▶ Chap. 5), close collaboration with an expert gastrointestinal histopathologist should be sought for feedback on image interpretation. The possibility of simultaneous image interpretation and collaboration with histopathology may even be achieved using modern telecommunication systems.

Time requirements for confocal imaging have been studied in a prospective trial for colonoscopy. By adding both confocal endomicroscopy and chromoendoscopy to videoendoscopy, total examination time increased from an average of 31 min to 42 min in surveillance of patients with longstanding ulcerative colitis [1]. As with every examination technique, time requirements for confocal endomicroscopy are highly dependent on the expert status of the endoscopist.

4.5   Fluorescent Agents

Confocal endomicroscopy uses stimulated light emission and relies on the application of fluorescent agents. Fluorescein, acriflavine, tetracycline and, to a lesser extent, cresyl violet are compatible with currently available laser light and filtering options and have been studied in animals and human subjects. In most studies, intravenous fluorescein sodium or topical acriflavine hydrochloride were evaluated (◘ Fig. 4.7).

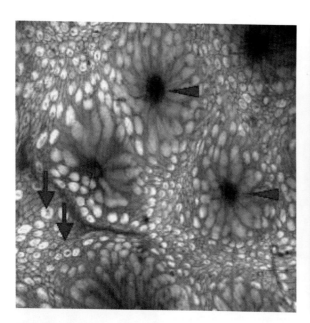
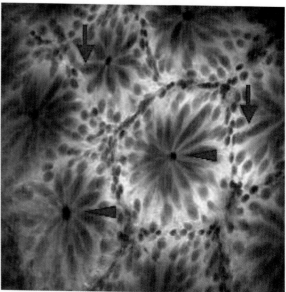

◘ **Fig. 4.7.** Superficial optical sections through normal colon mucosa. *Left panel*: Topical application of acriflavine hydrochloride stains nuclei of colonic goblet cells and absorptive cells around the crypt opening (*arrowheads*). Goblet cells can be identified by the bottle-neck opening of the mucin inclusion (*arrows*). *Right panel*: After fluorescein injection, the cytoplasm of the cells is highlighted, while the nuclei cannot be directly visualised. Mucin inside the goblet cells remains black (*arrows*). Capillaries are not seen at superficial sections of the epithelial layer

Fluorescein sodium is an inexpensive contrast agent that has been used clinically by ophthalmologists for fluorescence angiography for several decades. Fluorescein emits light at wavelengths of 520–530 nm during stimulation by laser light at wavelengths of 465–490 nm. Thus, the fluorescein dye is excited by blue light and emits light that appears yellowish-green. Fluorescein is rapidly metabolised by the liver into fluorescein monoglucoronide and is excreted by the kidney. No dose adjustment is necessary for renal- or hepatic-impaired patients. In general, only one vial of fluorescein is injected per patient. Adverse events have only rarely been reported [2]. These include allergic reactions with a drop in blood pressure or cardiac rhythm abnormalities (0.6%), nausea (3.5%), or local complications such as extravasation and/or thrombophlebitis (0.16 %) [11, 12]. A transient yellowish colouring of the skin and urine for up to 6 h occurs regularly. No other side effects of intravenous fluorescein sodium have been documented in human confocal endomicroscopy cases.

During confocal endomicroscopy, 5 ml of 10% fluorescein sodium is injected intravenously. Its distribution throughout the entire tissue within seconds after intravenous administration results in a bright contrast over the whole optical range of the z-axis. Fluorescein provides a good impression of the tissue architecture by highlighting vessels, cells and connective tissue. Nuclei cannot be visualised in most cells directly due to the pharmacological properties of fluorescein. However, nuclear configuration may be derived from the intracellular dye distribution. Fluorescein wash-out start 20 min after injection, but examination times up to 60 min are possible with good image quality. A second injection of 5 ml is possible and does not appear to increase the rate of complications. Since fluorescein is excreted by the kidneys, renal impairment as marked by elevated creatinine levels is considered a relative contraindication for intravenous fluorescein use [13].

Acriflavine hydrochloride stains the nuclei and also helps visualise the cytoplasm to a lesser extent. It therefore gives an excellent impression of the tissue, and in animal studies it has been shown to reliably predict cellular features known from conventional histology that predict neoplasia, such as an altered nuclear-to-cytoplasm ratio and chromatin condensation. However, theoretical concerns have been raised about the use of acriflavine. Since nuclear enrichment might indicate biochemical interaction, even topical use of acriflavine carries a potential risk of mutagenicity. Originally, acriflavine was developed as an antifungal agent and it is still frequently used in topical antiseptics with no carcinogenic effects reported so far after many decades of use. However, use of acriflavine should be carefully considered, especially when screening for intraepithelial neoplasias or cancer. Cresyl violet, an alternative agent with fluorescence, might overcome these concerns but has not been tested in large human trials of in vivo confocal imaging. Acriflavine hydrochloride is applied topically by using 10–50 ml of a 0.02% solution via a conventional spraying catheter. Dye spraying results in staining of cell layers close to the tissue surface only (i.e. superficial 50 μm). Since fluorescein allows subsurface imaging over the complete optical sectioning capability of the device, it has been found to be more appropriate for most indications [7–10].

References

1. Kiesslich R, Burg J, Vieth M et al (2004) Confocal laser endoscopy for diagnosing intraepithelial neoplasias and colorectal cancer in vivo. Gastroenterology 127:706–713
2. Thong PS, Olivo M, Kho KW, Zheng W, Mancer K, Harris M, Soo KC (2007) Laser confocal endomicroscopy as a novel technique for fluorescence diagnostic imaging of the oral cavity. J Biomed Opt 12:014007
3. Hoffman A, Goetz M, Vieth M, Galle PR, Neurath MF, Kiesslich R (2006) Confocal laser endomicroscopy: technical status and current indications. Endoscopy 38:1275–1283
4. Kitabatake S, Niwa Y, Miyahara R, Ohashi A, Matsuura T, Iguchi Y, Shimoyama Y, Nagasaka T, Maeda O, Ando T, Ohmiya N, Itoh A, Hirooka Y, Goto H (2006) Confocal endomicroscopy for the diagnosis of gastric cancer in vivo. Endoscopy 38:1110–1114
5. Kakeji Y, Yamaguchi S, Yoshida D, Tanoue K, Ueda M, Masunari A, Utsunomiya T, Imamura M, Honda H, Maehara Y, Hashizume M (2006) Development and assessment of morphologic criteria for diagnosing gastric cancer using confocal endomicroscopy: an ex vivo and in vivo study. Endoscopy 38:886–890
6. Hurlstone DP, Sanders DS (2006) Recent advances in chromoscopic colonoscopy and endomicroscopy. Curr Gastroenterol Rep 8:409–415
7. Goetz M, Hoffman A, Galle PR, Neurath MF, Kiesslich R (2006) Confocal laser endoscopy: new approach to the early diagnosis of tumors of the esophagus and stomach. Future Oncol 2:469–476
8. Kiesslich R, Gossner L, Goetz M, Dahlmann A, Vieth M, Stolte M, Hoffman A, Jung M, Nafe B, Galle PR, Neurath MF (2006) In vivo histology of Barrett's esophagus and associated neoplasia by confocal laser endomicroscopy. Clin Gastroenterol Hepatol 4:979–987
9. Kiesslich R, Hoffman A, Goetz M, Biesterfeld S, Vieth M, Galle PR, Neurath MF (2006) In vivo diagnosis of collagenous colitis by confocal endomicroscopy. Gut 55:591–592

10. Kiesslich R, Goetz M, Schneider C et al (2005) Confocal endomicroscopy as a novel method to diagnose colitis associated neoplasias in ulcerative colitis: a prospective randomized trial [abstract]. Digestive Disease Week 2005. Gastroenterology 128:A35 [Suppl 2]

11. Kwiterovich KA, Maguire MG, Murphy RP, Schachat AP, Bressler NM, Bressler SB, Fine SL (1991) Frequency of adverse systemic reactions after fluorescein angiography. Results of a prospective study. Ophthalmology 98:1139–1142

12. Pacuriariu RI (1982) Low incidence of side effects following intravenous fluorescein angiography. Ann Ophtalmol 14:32–36

13. Polglase AL, McLaren W, Skinner SA, Kiesslich R, Neurath MF, Delaney PM (2005) A fluorescence confocal endomicroscope for in vivo microscopy of the upper- and lower-GI tract. Gastrointest Endosc 62:686–695

4

The Technique of Confocal Laser Endomicroscopy from the Perspective of a New User

Marcia I. Canto

Key concepts:
- Hands on training and clinical practice are required for mastery in endomicroscopy.
- The technique is relatively easy to perform after structured training.
- Artefacts noted during endomicroscopy may consist of motion and image artefacts.

5.1 Introduction

Confocal laser endomicroscopy (CLE) is a valuable new technique for obtaining in vivo, real-time histology. As with any new endoscopic technique, training and practice are required for mastery. The specifics of the confocal endomicroscope are described in ► Chap. 4 (◘ Fig. 4.1).

Important features for the new user include the use of button 4, located on the back-left of the hand piece, which causes the confocal imaging direction to return to the 'home' position approximately 10 µm below the surface. This is a useful function if you get »lost« and are unsure about whether you are in the superficial or deep mucosa. Button 3 is used frequently during endomicroscopic imaging to move the scanning direction one plane up or down, depending upon the direction of imaging. It is also important to remember that the confocal imaging window is located 5 mm to the left of the biopsy channel. This is important for obtaining targeted biopsies after endomicroscopic imaging. Furthermore, it is important to point out that videoendoscopic and endomicroscopic images are displayed simultaneously during CLE (◘ Fig. 5.1). Confocal images are captured with the help of a foot pedal.

5.2 Preparation for Endomicroscopic Imaging

5.2.1 Entering Case Data and Imaging Sites

When the endomicroscopy software boots up, there will be self-explanatory choices presented to you to enter case information into the computer. Patient information, performing physician, date, indication and relevant clinical notes can all be entered and saved. A list of body sites to be used during confocal imaging can be created and saved. The list is located on the right side of the screen, and specific sites may be chosen and moved to the 'selected sites' list on the left of the screen by using the arrow key in the middle of the screen. You can create body sites such as »oesophagus«, »stomach«, »duodenum«, »right colon«, transverse colon«, »left colon«, and »rectum«, as well as name abnormalities such as »lesion 1«, »mass«, »polyp«, »Barrett's oesophagus«, etc. Alternatively, it may be useful to sequentially number confocal sites (such as »site_01, site_02, site_03«, etc.) and simply record the organ site, lesion type, and endoscopic diagnosis in clinical notes. Once a site is created in the list, it will be available for subsequent imaging cases. Each site selected will create a specific image folder, and all images acquired when a

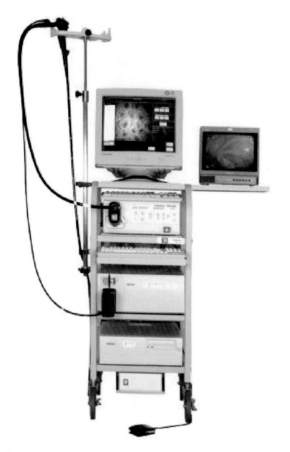

Fig. 5.1. Endomicroscopy system. On the *right monitor* the endoscopic image is visible, whereas the *left monitor* shows the endomicroscopic image at the same time

particular site is selected are stored in that folder. This is important for later review of images, image retrieval and archiving of images.

5.2.2 Study the Control Screen

During endomicroscopic imaging, you will need to control the scanning function of the endomicroscope. Hence, it is important to understand the various functions of the touch screen panel (Fig. 5.2). Remember that the touch screen controls may not work with a gloved hand. You can prepare for CLE using the touch screen without gloves but you may need to manipulate the control screen during the procedure with the keyboard mouse or have an assistant make changes on the touch screen for you.

At the top right corner of the control screen, the direction of optical scanning from the surface of the mucosa will be indicated by an up or down arrow in the top section governing »Depth« (Fig. 5.2, yellow arrow 1). The laser power is controlled by the function »Laser Control« (Fig. 5.2, yellow arrow 2). If image brightness needs to be increased during the procedure, you can decrease the laser rather than change the default settings for the brightness and gamma settings during endomicroscopic imaging.

When you are a new user, set the scanning rate (Scan Mode Control, Fig. 5.2, blue arrow) for »slower« (1.8 frames/s or 1024 × 1024 pixels) to allow enough time for examination of each confocal image. Endoscopists who are more experienced with confocal image interpretation may set the scanning rate to »faster« or 1.6 frames/s (1024 × 512 pixels) for more efficient optical biopsy.

At the bottom left portion of the control screen (»Site Control«, green arrow), you can select the body site location where the confocal images will be stored from the site list you created prior to starting the procedure (select »next«) or add a new site label by using the »Modify Site List« function.

5.2.3 Check the Laser and Calibrate

Make sure the laser is turned on by choosing the default mid position on the control screen (Fig. 5.2, yellow arrow 1). A blue laser light that is actively scanning should also be visible on the tip of the endoscope. The control panel should also indicate that the endomicroscope is not on »Standby« mode and the laser power should be approximately 500 µW. If the laser power appears very low, there may be a connection problem between the laser plug of the endoscope and the confocal computer. Restarting the setup process after reconnecting the plug will typically return the laser to normal power. Once you are done with setting up the case on the computer, calibrate the laser by pressing button 4 once. The upper right hand part of the touch panel control screen should indicate that calibration is ongoing by showing an hourglass. Place the fluorescein-impregnated calibrating cloth onto the confocal imaging window. You should see an image on the screen of bright and dark cloth fibres. Make sure that there is a confocal image uniformly seen throughout the square box (475 × 475 µm). It is also useful to capture one to two images during the calibration, which may be useful for comparison if any image quality problems are

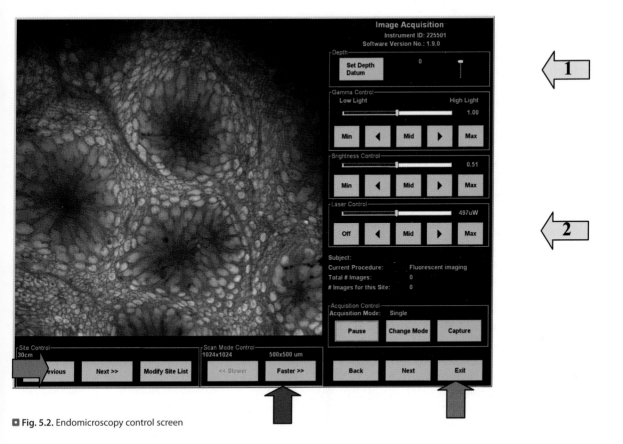

Fig. 5.2. Endomicroscopy control screen

noted during the procedure or during image review, such as blurred or dark images.

5.2.4 Obtaining Informed Consent

In the United States, fluorescein sodium is approved by the Food and Drug Administration (FDA) for ophthalmological procedures such as retinal angiography. Currently, its use in CLE would be considered off-label use of fluorescein sodium. In the near future, there will be FDA approval for the combination of intravenous fluorescein and CLE. A discussion with the patient about the risks and benefits of performing CLE with fluorescein should be completed prior to the procedure, just as is done for ancillary endoscopic imaging procedures such as endoscopic ultrasound. Standardised written discharge instructions related to CLE should be created and given to the patient to take home and should be reviewed by the nurse prior to the procedure.

Intravenous fluorescein sodium has been used in retinal angiography or angioscopy of the fundus and iris vasculature for many years and is very safe. It causes yellow discoloration of the skin, which fades after 6–12 h. However, urine fluorescence can continue up to 36 h. Make sure you or your staff inquire specifically about the use of contact lenses, which may be discoloured by fluorescein. Contact lenses should be removed prior to the procedure. Mild adverse reactions of fluorescein sodium can also include nausea (2–20% of patients) and vomiting (0–7% of patients). Extravasation of fluorescein during injection is rare (<3% of injections in ophthalmological studies), but can cause superficial thrombophlebitis, with no to mild discomfort. If a large amount of fluorescein extravasates, cellulitis or tissue necrosis can occur. Intra-arterial injection has been reported but is rare, but no serious sequelae have been described. All patients receiving intravenous fluorescein sodium for confocal CLE will have a peripheral i.v. placed, reducing the risk of intra-arterial injection. Skin eruptions have been described in 0–1% of patients; these can be treated with diphenhydramine. Rare cases of vasovagal syncope have been reported. Cardiovascular complications are reported with an incidence of one in 5300 patients and pulmonary complications one in 3800. Use in patients with known allergy to fluorescein sodium should be avoided, as there have been case reports of anaphylaxis.

5.3 General Technique of Confocal Endomicroscopic Imaging

Perform a routine videoendoscopic evaluation prior to endomicroscopic imaging. The endoscopic in vivo diagnosis should always be a composite of the standard videoendoscopic findings and the endomicroscopic images.

There are five components of endomicroscopic imaging:

1. Targeting of a lesion or area of interest for imaging and achieving contact with the confocal window
2. Acquisition of a stable position for imaging and minimising artefact
3. Performance of confocal endomicroscopic imaging
4. Interpretation of images
5. Assessment of the need for targeted biopsies

5.3.1 Targeting of a Lesion or Area

To facilitate endomicroscopic imaging of a targeted lesion, place the target in the left lower corner of the endoscopic view. This corresponds to the location of the confocal endomicroscope imaging window (◘ Fig. 5.1).

5.3.2 Achieving Contact of the Confocal Window with the Mucosa

The general goal is to manoeuvre the endomicroscope tip to allow en face gentle contact of the confocal imaging window with the mucosal or lesion surface. Sufficient contact of the entire confocal lens with the mucosa is indicated by the presence of an image filling the entire square of the viewing portion of the monitor. In general, you will need to tip down, torque the scope slightly anticlockwise and push the tip gently towards the seven o'clock position of the endoscopic view to achieve sufficient contact with the mucosa. If you see the blue laser light on the mucosa in the standard videoendoscopic screen, you have not achieved contact of the mucosa with the confocal imaging window.

5.3.3 Acquiring a Stable Position

First of all, stabilise the endomicroscope by pinning the endoscope shaft to the stretcher with the front of your thigh. This will minimise proximal and distal movement of the endoscope. If gentle pressure does not result in an adequate stable image, apply constant suction by keeping your finger on the suction valve. Avoid releasing suction during imaging as this will cause motion artefact.

5.3.4 Performing Endomicroscopic Imaging

Fluorescein sodium is the main contrast agent used in confocal endomicroscopy. Inject 5 ml of 10% fluorescein sodium (sterile solution) into the vein only when you are ready to start imaging because its onset of action is within 7–14 s and its duration of action is about 45 min (average 30–60 min). The rapidity of onset and duration of action may vary in some patients due to body habitus and other factors. In general, only one vial of fluorescein is injected per patient.

5.3.5 Planning the Anatomical Sites for Endomicroscopic Imaging

In the upper gastrointestinal tract, the least number of blood vessels are seen in the oesophagus, followed by the stomach and the duodenum. Hence, right after fluorescein injection, we prefer to image the oesophagus and leave the duodenum for last because of the marked brightness of the latter images. When confocal endomicroscopy is performed in the colon, imaging generally starts after the caecum or terminal ileum is reached.

Similar to endoscopic ultrasound (EUS), shift your focus from the endoscopic image to the endomicroscopic images displayed on the monitor. There are four key movements to make after you gain a stable position with little motion artefact. Firstly, change the direction of laser scanning towards or beneath the mucosal surface (i.e. moving towards or away from the surface by clicking button 3 once on the endoscope head (◘ Fig. 5.1) to allow optical sectioning of the superficial and deep mucosa.

Each click results in a 10–15 µm change in the imaging plane. If you would like to scan quickly and sequentially in one direction keep button 3 pressed; this will result in sequential generation of images until you release the button. If you want to remain at the same level within the mucosa, the laser will continue to scan by default and to »refresh« the image.

Secondly, optimise the images. If the image appears too bright or too dark, make adjustments to laser power (◘ Fig. 5.2) rather than to brightness on the control panel by moving the cursor to the left or right. The image may be very bright in the middle part of the mucosa right after injection due to the higher number of capillaries. On the other hand, the images of the gastric mucosa may generally appear slightly darker and the laser power should be increased when imaging in the stomach.

During CLE, you may also note that there is a solid line below the up arrow or above the down arrow on the depth control panel in the right upper portion of the control screen (yellow arrow 1), which indicates that the scanning plane is at the very top of the mucosa, or at the very bottom of the imaging range (at about 250 µm).

5.3.6 Identifying and Minimising Image Artefact

There are two general types of artefact noted during CLE (◘ Table 5.1). The most common is motion artefact (◘ Fig. 5.3). This appears as wavy lines and blurring of images. It is more commonly seen during imaging in the oesophagus and least evident during rectal imaging. Motion artefact is caused by patient movement, endoscope movement, tip movement, the patient's respiratory movements and beating heart, and normal gastrointestinal motility. Hence, motion artefact can be seen in approximately 60–70% of all oesophageal endomicroscopic images but in only about 25–30% of all colon and rectal images. If motion artefact is not avoidable due to multiple contractions and cardiac pulsations, beginners can capture confocal images at the »faster« rate and review these images before changing position in the GI tract.

The other type of artefact seen in confocal endomicroscopy is image artefact. Image artefact can be caused by contamination with blood, extravasated fluorescein, or stool on the confocal lens. Avoid suctioning friable or inflamed mucosa because the blood will extravasate and the fluorescein will cause artefactual brightness on the mucosal surface. If you decide to perform mucosal biopsies, do this as the last part of the procedure after all confocal imaging is complete or perform a biopsy of an area distal and distant from the next imaging site. The blood may contaminate other mucosal areas and cause image artefact from fluorescence. In the colon, frequently wash any residual stool away before it dries on the confocal image window. The confocal window can also be gently

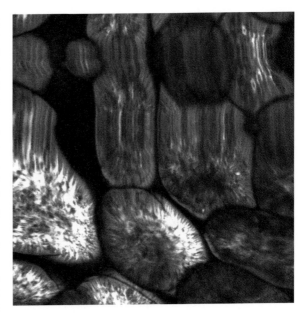

◘ **Fig. 5.3.** Motion artefact

◘ **Table 5.1.** Types of confocal endomicroscopic artefacts

Types	Causes
Motion	– Unstable endoscope position – Patient movement – Gastrointestinal motility
Image	
– Bright splotches on the image – Dark splotches on the image – Uniformly dark confocal image – Lack of a confocal image	Imaging on folds – Blood with fluorescein – Residual stool or undigested material – Absent or low level of fluorescein, laser power too low – Processor on standby; fluorescein was not injected

wiped along clean areas of the colonic mucosa to remove stool particles. When imaging in the rectum, material on the lens can be removed by withdrawing the endomicroscope and wiping the confocal lens with gauze.

An additional type of image artefact is caused by imaging on a fold, which results in artefactual darkening of cells and may incorrectly suggest the possibility of neoplasia. Incomplete filling of the screen with tissue, crypts or villi that change angulation in the same image, and large white areas or partially blurred images on the screen can suggest that imaging is occurring on a fold. Repositioning the endoscope by gently turning the wheels and applying gentle pressure to the mucosa may relieve this type of artefact. Before concluding that neoplasia is present or absent, several stable images of the same area at varying depths should be obtained. An unstable endoscope position leads to motion artefacts, where horizontal lines become visible and disturb image interpretation.

5.3.7   Limitations

The current fluorescence agent fluorescein does not allow routine imaging of nuclei; therefore, mild or low-grade dysplasia that is based primarily on changes of nuclei cannot be reliably diagnosed. On the other hand, high-grade dysplasia and cancer can be readily and accurately diagnosed due to a combination of distortion of architecture and alteration of cellular morphology, hyperchromasia, increased vascularity, distortion of blood vessels bridging crypts, and leakage from capillaries.

The penetration depth of confocal CLE is limited (about $250\,\mu m$ deep from the mucosal surface) to the superficial and deep mucosa. Hence, it is not suitable for staging of cancers.

5.4   Image Annotation, Export, Archive and Review

5.4.1   Annotating Images

Annotation of endomicroscopic images can be performed during or after the procedure. Annotate an image by moving to the image review screen by pressing »Next« (◲ Fig. 5.2, orange arrow), then using the »Add Note« features. This will put a tag on the particular image you select, and you can then add detailed description in text.

5.4.2   Saving and Exporting Images

After the procedure, you can review the images from any patient or any date by sorting by name or procedure date. If you would like to export all the images of a patient from one procedure, the images can be exported to a CD using the 'format CD' and 'export' functions. Zipped files of each confocal case can also be exported for backup. The 'save as' function can also be used to save individual or collections of confocal images. The system defaults to highlight or select all folders (confocal imaging sites). You can then select »save as«, and high-quality jpeg images may be saved to a particular computer location. Ideally, all procedure images should be archived on a separate hard drive. We find network drives to be particularly more useful than external USB drives or exporting to CD, as they are routinely backed up and can be accessed for review or insertion into Microsoft Powerpoint or word processing documents using the Internet.

5.4.3   Reviewing Images

Image review is integral to learning endomicroscopy image interpretation. We strongly encourage you to review confocal images soon after the procedure to continue improving your understanding of confocal image interpretation and to correlate these images with the corresponding mucosal biopsies on a routine basis (such as twice a month). You may also wish to track your learning process for confocal endomicroscopy. Several components to examine include the time needed for a confocal endomicroscopy procedure, the number of images taken per case, the proportion of images that have little to no image artefact (which may vary by site), and the proportion of images that have useful information.

In conclusion, endomicroscopy is a highly examiner dependent endoscopic tool. Thorough knowledge about the endomicroscopic system, contrast agents, examination technique and histology is mandatory to speed up the learning curve. Intensive interaction with the pathologist also helps to improve the diagnostic yield. However, confocal imaging can be learned by endoscopists, and interpretation of in vivo histology during ongoing endoscopy might help to reduce the number of biopsies and to target biopsies to relevant changes.

Microarchitecture of the Normal Gut Seen with Conventional Histology and Endomicroscopy

Michael Vieth, Ralf Kiesslich, Steven Thomas, Peter Delaney

Key concepts:
- Endomicroscopy allows to access the mucosal layer of the esophagus, stomach, small and large bowel.
- In vivo imaging leads to a new understanding of the healthy and diseased GI tract.
- Conventional histology and endomicroscopy are supplementary techniques.

6.1 Introduction

For ex vivo histological examination of the gastrointestinal tract, fractions of an organ or small pieces of tissue are needed. Several steps are used in the fixation, staining, and mounting process to ensure production of good-quality histology on glass slides. The most frequently used stain in routine histology is the haematoxylin and eosin (H&E) stain. The most frequently used tissue-staining methods are shown in ◘ Table 6.1. The final histopathological diagnosis is always based on examination of the whole sample and the structure and architecture of that sample. In cytology, single cells and nuclei are used for making a diagnosis, so staining procedures in cytology are much faster and easier to perform.

Endomicroscopy makes it possible to assess the mucosal layer in vivo. Living cells can be observed; this leads to functional analysis and offers the unique possibility of seeing in vivo the architecture of the mucosal layer. Confocal images are displayed as grey scale images. Currently, two different contrast agents are used that allow fluorescence imaging.

Intravenous fluorescein is distributed throughout the body and the mucosal layer of the gut can be observed over the whole range of the endomicroscope's dynamic imaging plane ranging from the surface up to 250 µm deep. However, nuclei cannot be readily identified using fluorescein. Therefore, tissue analysis is focused more on pattern recognition than on analysis of nuclei architecture. Acriflavine-aided endomicroscopy leads to a strong labelling of nuclei and cell membranes. It is a topical and absorptive dye. Therefore, only the upper third of the mucosal layer can be displayed endomicroscopically. The two different staining agents can be used singly or in combination.

6.2 General Structure and Components of the Gastrointestinal Tract

In general, the tubular gastrointestinal tract can be subdivided into four major parts:
1. oesophagus
2. stomach
3. small bowel
4. colon

Each of these segments is separated from the other by a muscular sphincter. Furthermore, the epithelial lining of

◨ **Table 6.1.** Frequently used conventional staining methods in histology and cytology

Method	Purpose	Example
Haematoxylin and eosin (H&E)	staining of nuclei and cytoplasm	routine stain, all slides
Giemsa stain	cytological details (nuclei, cytoplasm)	haematology, e.g. lymph nodes, bone marrow
Warthin-Starry silver stain	contrast enhancement of nuclei	visualisation of bacteria such as *Helicobacter* spp.
van-Gieson's stain	staining of elastic and collagen fibres	vessel walls, liver biopsies, mesenchymal tumours
Gomori's silver stain	agyrophilic fibres	bone marrow, lymph nodes
PAS reaction	neutral mucopolysaccharides	mucinous adenocarcinoma, signet ring cell carcinoma
PAS-alcian blue	neutral and acid mucopolysaccharides	mucinous adenocarcinoma, menisci, mesothelioma
Turnbull	haemosiderin	residue of prior bleeding, bone marrow, trauma
Congo Red stain	amyloid	primary and secondary amyloidosis
Ziehl-Neelson stain	acid-resistant bacteria	bacterial infections (mycobacteria and other)
Gram's stain	gram-positive bacteria	bacterial infections (*Staphylococcus* and other)
Grocott's stain	fungal structures	mycosis (aspergillosis, moniliasis)
Pappenheim's stain	cytological differentiation	haematology and cytological preparations (ascites)
Papanicolaou's stain	cytological differentiation	gynaecological cytology

the gastrointestinal tract changes in an abrupt manner at the junction of each segment of the GI tract, such as the change between the squamous epithelium of the oesophagus and the columnar epithelium of the stomach.

Although the basic architecture is comparable in all regions of the gastrointestinal tract, the functional and structural differences of each segment are important for digestion and passage of food and fluids. The chief features seen in each part of the GI tract include the mucosal layer;, a submucosal layer which is separated from the mucosal layer by the muscularis mucosa; the muscularis propria, which contains circular and longitudinal muscle compartments, and the serosa, which includes subserosal connective tissue.

The mucosal layer always consists of an epithelial lining with a basement membrane and connective tissue containing mostly lymphocytes and plasma cells (together called the lamina propria), lined by a thin layer of smooth muscle fibres called the muscularis mucosa. This is followed by another layer of connective tissue, the submucosal layer, which again contains immunocompetent cells (but to a lesser degree than the lamina propria), mid-sized blood vessels, and lymphatic vessels. The adjacent layer is built by the thick muscularis propria that consists of two layers – the outer longitudinal and inner circular bundles of smooth muscle. Bundles of smooth muscle cells are connected to each other by nexuses to ensure regular contractions during food and fluid passage.

6.3 Mucosal Layer

6.3.1 Oesophagus

The mucosa that lines the oesophagus is a non-keratinised, stratified squamous epithelium (◨ Fig. 6.1) that provides protection from physical abrasion by ingested food. The squamous epithelium consists of a variable number of cell layers, which exhibit transition from a cuboidal basal layer to a more flattened surface layer. The nuclei near the luminal surface are also more flattened. The interface between the surface epithelium and the underlying supporting tissue is marked by a non-cellular structure known as the basement membrane (BM). The BM provides structural support for the epithelial cells from the underlying lamina propria (LP). In human beings, the epithelium is quite thick (300–500 μm) and is constantly renewed by mitosis in the basal cells. As they migrate towards the lumen, they become progressively polygonal and more flattened and are eventually desquamated at the epithelial surface.

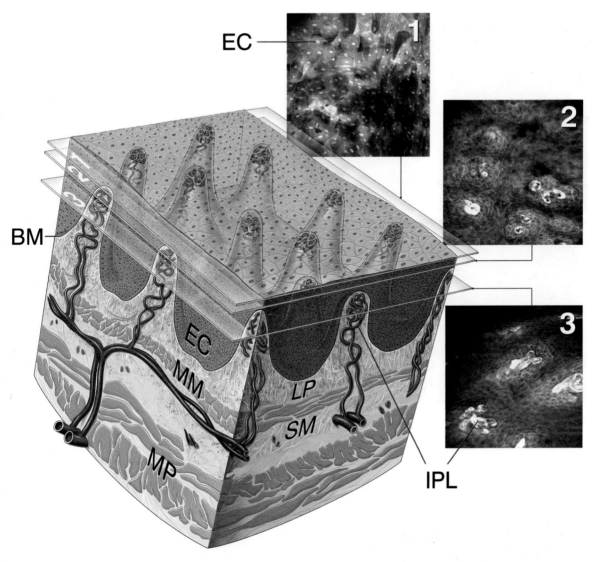

Fig. 6.1. Microarchitecture of the distal oesophagus. *EC* Epithelial cells; *BM* basement membrane; *LP* lamina propria; *MM* lamina muscularis mucosae; *SM* submucosa; *MP* lamina muscularis propria; *IPL* intrapapillary loops

The epithelial cells are kept moist by glandular secretions from (submucosal) proper oesophageal glands. The muscularis mucosa delineates the mucosal layer from the submucosa. The epithelium can be easily differentiated from the adjacent tissue by the presence of the basal cell layer that is composed of relatively small, uniform hyperchromatic cells (❏ Fig. 6.2). All proliferation and regeneration of the oesophageal squamous epithelium derives from this basal layer. During inflammatory or regenerative processes this layer is significantly thickened and can

reach more than half of the total epithelial thickness. In most cases of inflammation, such as in reflux disease, the basal layer is thickened and the space between the cells is widened; this is called intercellular dilatation (❏ Fig. 6.3). It is believed that refluate or other irritants can reach the free nerve endings of the oesophageal epithelium and cause pain by filtering through the intercellular dilatations. Intercellular dilatations of more than 5 μm (about the diameter of a lymphocyte) are considered marked changes, whereas minimal changes are considered to start from 1.2 μm inter-

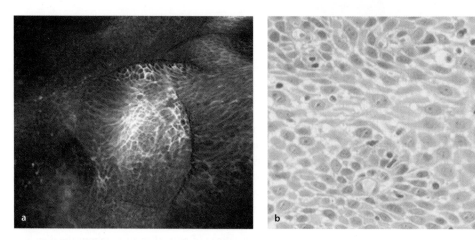

◪ **Fig. 6.2a–e.** Endomicroscopy of the oesophagus. **a** White-light endoscopic view of the distal oesophagus. The whitish squamous epithelium (*arrow*) can be readily identified and differentiated from columnar epithelium. **b** Conventional histology of the normal squamous epithelium of the distal oesophagus. Squamous epithelial cells with nuclei can be seen (*orange arrow*). Papillae exiting from the lamina propria into the epithelial layer contain intrapapillary capillaries (*blue arrow*). **c** Endomicroscopic image of surface squamous epithelium with visible nuclei (*arrow*) after acriflavine staining. **d** Intrapapillary loops (*arrow*) and squamous epithelium in the upper portion of the mucosa. **e** Non-erosive reflux disease with dilated intercellular spaces and increased vasculature (*arrow*)

◪ **Fig. 6.3a,b.** Non-erosive reflux disease. **a** Endomicroscopic image (fluorescein staining) of squamous epithelium after acid exposure in a patient with non erosive reflux disease. A marked dilatation of intercellular spaces is visible and the underlying fluorescence shines through the spaces (*arrow*). **b** Corresponding conventional histology with dilatation of intercellular spaces

cellular dilatations. Short indentations of soft tissue into the squamous epithelium are called epithelial papillae. In cases of ongoing proliferation or inflammatory reactions these papillae are elongated and can reach more than 90% of the total epithelial thickness. In normal tissue, these papillae are not elongated more than 10–20% of the total epithelial thickness. After therapy with proton pump inhibitors all of these reflux-associated cellular changes are reversible.

The cells in the more apical layer of the squamous epithelium, the stratum spinosum, contain larger nuclei with less hyperchromasia compared with the basal cells. As cells approach the apical layer of the squamous epithelium they change shape and become flattened. This fact is useful in cytology for estimating the origin of a certain cell.

6.3.2 Endomicroscopic Imaging of Normal Oesophageal Mucosa

The mucosa of the oesophagus consists of a non-keratinised squamous epithelium. The structures imaged en face using confocal endomicroscopy change with the depth of the focal plane and with the fluorescent dye used for image contrast. Topical application of acriflavine (0.05%) stains the cell nuclei of the surface epithelium and enables imaging of the polygonal surface cell layers (◘ image 1 in Fig. 6.1). Following the intravenous administration of fluorescein sodium (5–10 ml of a 10% solution), it is possible to visualise the capillary loops of the oesophageal papillae and the surrounding epithelial cells (◘ images 2 and 3 in Fig. 6.1). The papillae are tall invaginations of the basement membrane that are rich in nerves and blood vessels. Erythrocytes in the lumen of the vessels do not take up the contrast agent and therefore appear as dark cells amidst the fluorescent plasma. Optical penetration is such that various cell layers can be seen, with squamous cells appearing larger nearer the surface, where they are more flattened. The basal cells are seen adjacent to the papillae, but the deepest basal cells are rarely observed, except in situations where the overall thickness of the epithelium may be reduced. In such cases, it is sometimes possible to observe the underlying sub-epithelial stroma including the larger, more linearly arranged arterioles and venules, which connect to the papillary capillary loops. The barrier function of this epithelium also greatly influences the microscopy – intravenously injected fluorescein sodium will permeate most of the epithelial cell matrix but is prevented from permeating the top 10-20 µm where the barrier function is normal. This may be altered when barrier function is compromised, allowing more fluorescein to permeate more superficially, or even to reach the surface. Likewise, topically applied agents do not generally permeate beyond the most superficial squamous cells. Fluorescein-aided endomicroscopy highlights mainly intrapapillary capillaries (loops) within the squamous epithelium, whereas acriflavine-aided endomicroscopy can be used to highlight specifically single squamous epithelium including nuclei, cytoplasm and cell membrane.

6.3.3 Stomach

The stomach can be subdivided into three or even four parts: the most distal part, the antrum, consists of foveolar epithelium and basal mucoid glands. The proximal part of the stomach, the corpus or body, typically contains a small apical portion of foveolar epithelium, followed by glandular epithelium specific to the body, which includes the chief cells and the parietal cells. The two remaining parts of the stomach are composed of a kind of transitional epithelium. One part is the intermediate zone, where the antral mucosa changes into corpus mucosa, and the second is the cardia, which is the ill-defined zone between the distal oesophagus and the proximal stomach. It is now clear that the cardia type of mucosa is not metaplastic per se, but is often only a few millimetres long and can enlarge with age.

The epithelium of the stomach can be further subdivided. The apical foveolar epithelium can be divided into the gastric pits, which are nearest the lumen; the neck of the glands, found within the gastric regeneration zone; and the basal body of the glands, which reaches down to the muscularis mucosa. In the normal stomach there are no neutrophilic granulocytes present and no large amounts of lymphocytes or plasma cells.

Viewed microscopically, the internal surface of the stomach wall appears honeycombed by small, irregular gastric pits approximately 0.2 mm in diameter (◘ Fig. 6.4). The base of each gastric pit receives several long, tubular gastric glands that extend deep into the lamina propria, as far as the muscularis mucosae. Although all the gastric glands are tubular, they vary in form and cellular composition in different parts of the stomach. A single-layered columnar epithelium covers the entire luminal surface, including the gastric pits. The interface between the surface epithelium and the underlying supporting tissue is marked by the non-cellular BM, which provides structural

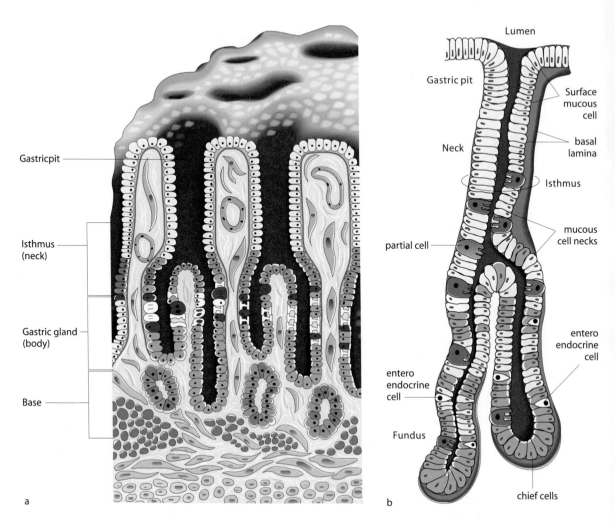

Fig. 6.4a,b. Microarchitecture of gastric glands. **a** Three-dimensional representation of the microstructure of the stomach. [12]. **b** Two-dimensional representation of a gastric pit and gastric gland of the stomach. [10]

support for the epithelial cells and constitutes a selective barrier to the passage of materials between the epithelium and the underlying supporting tissue (lamina propria).

Simple columnar mucus-secreting epithelium covers the entire surface of the stomach. The epithelium is composed of a continuous layer of surface mucous cells which release gastric mucus from their apical surfaces to form a protective, lubricant layer over the gastric lining. The epithelium commences abruptly in the cardia orifice, where there is a sudden transition from the stratified squamous epithelium of the oesophagus.

6.3.4 Endomicroscopic Imaging of Gastric Mucosa

The gastric mucosa of the stomach is comprised of a simple columnar epithelium that secretes mucus. When viewed microscopically following the i.v. administration of fluorescein sodium (5–10ml of a 10% solution), the internal surface of the stomach appears honeycombed by small, slightly irregular gastric glands, tiled with polygonal epithelial cells with a distinctive cobblestone appearance (◘ Figs. 6.5, 6.6). In the pyloric antrum (◘ images

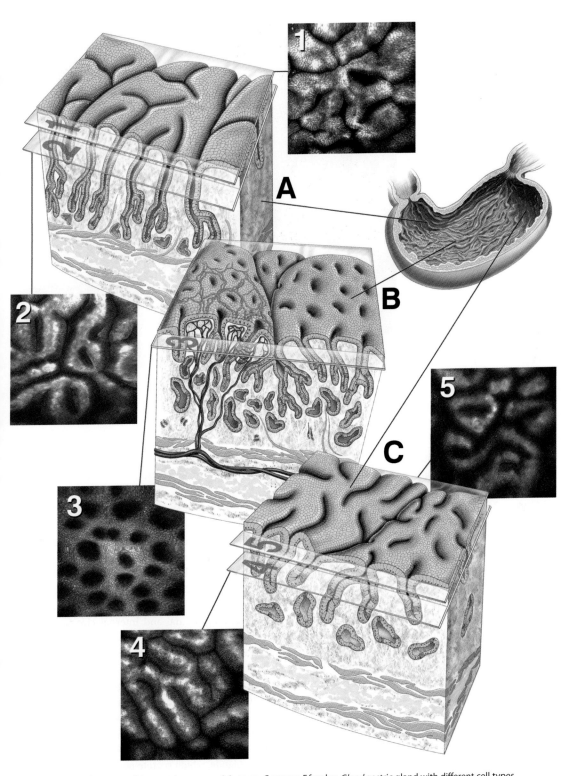

■ **Fig. 6.5.** Microarchitecture of the gastric mucosa. *A* Antrum, *C* corpus, *F* fundus, *Gland* gastric gland with different cell types

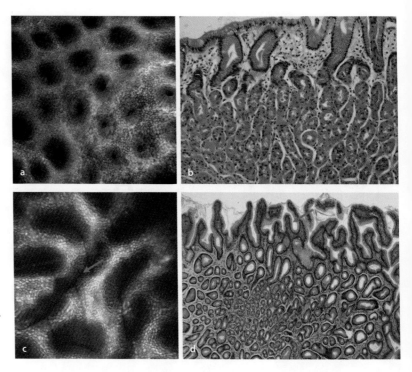

Fig. 6.6a–d. Endomicroscopy and conventional histology of normal gastric mucosa. **a** Endomicroscopy images gastric glands mainly on the upper third of the mucosal layer. The luminal openings of the gland can be readily identified (*arrow*). **b** Histology of the gastric corpus. Note the difference between the glands in the upper and lower portions of the mucosal layer. A luminal opening of a gastric gland as imaged with endomicroscopy is marked with an *arrow*. **c** The glands in the antrum are more elongated compared with the corpus (*arrow*). On the gastric surface a typical cobblestone appearance becomes visible, indicating gastric-type epithelium. This cobblestone appearance helps to differentiate gastric-type epithelium from a specialised type of metaplastic tissue within the distal oesophagus. **d** Corresponding conventional histology; the upper lumen of a single gland is marked with an *arrow*

1 and 2 in Fig. 6.5) and the fundus (■ images 4 and 5 in Fig. 6.5) there are many gastric folds, and the openings of the glands are long and more slit-like. In the corpus of the stomach (■ image 3 in Fig. 6.5), the glands are more round and regular in shape. At the surface, the columnar epithelium appears as a tiled mosaic of cells (■ images 1, 3 and 5 in Fig. 6.5). Just beneath the surface of the epithelial plane, the transverse alignment of epithelial cells lining the crypts is clearly visible. A differentiation between different types of cells (e.g. chief cells and parietal cells) is not possible endomicroscopically. Imaging further beneath the surface enables visualisation of the microvasculature within the lamina propria (■ images 2 and 4 in Fig. 6.4). The optical penetration is not as great in the stomach as in other GI mucosae, perhaps owing to differences in the cell matrix, mucus consistency and acidic environment, which for example suppress the fluorescence emission of some contrast agents, including fluorescein. However, as described above, both the epithelial cells and the subepithelial lamina propria and microvascular matrix can be observed clearly.

6.3.5 Small Bowel

The small bowel mucosa is composed of finger-like or leaf-like villi (■ Fig. 6.7). Villi of the small intestine are highly vascular, finger-like projections of the mucosal surface that significantly increase the absorptive area. Villi vary in density from 10 to 40/mm^2 and are generally 0.5–1.0 mm in length. Each villus contains a capillary network, a lymphatic vessel and smooth muscle fibres. The muscularis mucosa forms the base of the mucosa and has external longitudinal and internal circular layers of smooth muscle cells (■ Fig. 6.8).

The tubular glands or crypts are called the glands of Lieberkühn. The tunica propria contains lymphocytes and a few plasma cells. Lymphoid aggregates are unusual in the duodenum, while the ileum contains numerous Peyer's patches. Basal Paneth cells with eosinophilic antibacterial granules can be found in this layer. The submucosal layer in the duodenal bulb and parts of the duodenum contain Brunner's glands, which secrete neutral, viscous mucus to ensure neutralisation of acidic gastric contents.

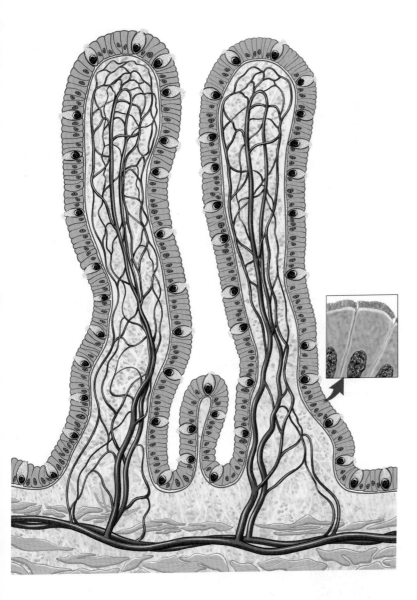

Fig. 6.7. Small bowel villi components

Typical small bowel mucosa contains numerous goblet cells, which interrupt the brush border. A few lymphocytes may be present in the epithelial layer but should not exceed 20–40/100 epithelial cells.

6.3.6 Endomicroscopic Imaging of Small Bowel Architecture

The mucosa of the small intestine contains thousands of finger-like projections (villi) consisting largely of a con-

nective tissue matrix covered by a single-layered columnar epithelium (⬛ Figs. 6.8, 6.9). When viewed microscopically following the i.v. administration of fluorescein sodium (5 ml of a 10% solution), the cells of the surface epithelium including the columnar epithelial cells (brightly fluorescent cells) and the mucus-containing goblet cells (dark circles) can be clearly observed. Folding of the villi frequently enables imaging in cross-section, when the capillaries contained within the core of the villi in the lamina propria can be observed (⬛ images 2 and 3 of Fig. 6.8). Villous intestinal epithelium appears to offer

6

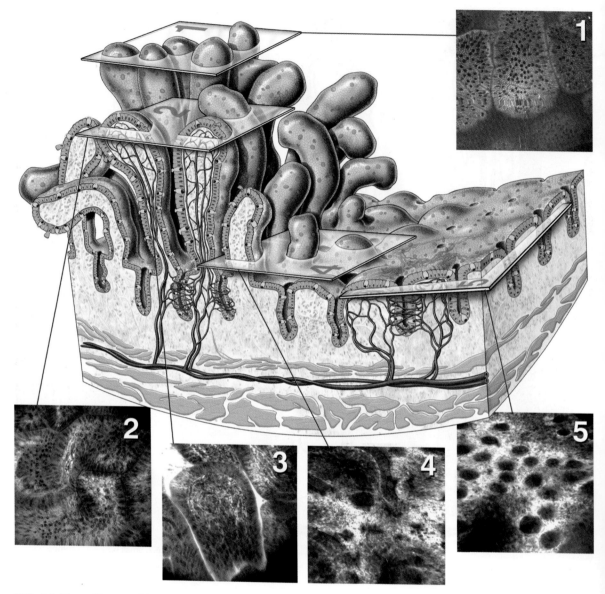

Fig. 6.8. Microarchitecture of the small bowel

good light penetration properties, with clear subsurface structures observable throughout most of the diameter of whole villi. However, the optical penetration is mostly insufficient to reveal the underlying glands amidst overlying healthy villi. In coeliac disease, however, the duodenal villi atrophy (■ image 4 of Fig. 6.8) or disappear completely (■ image 5 of Fig. 6.8), enabling visualisation of the underlying crypts at the base of the villi.

6.3.7 Colon

The mucosal surface of the colon is composed of thousands of crypts or glands orientated as straight tubular structures extending down to the muscularis mucosae. These glands are supported by a connective tissue matrix known as the lamina propria, which contains blood vessels, nerves, smooth muscle, collagen and elastin. The epithelium of

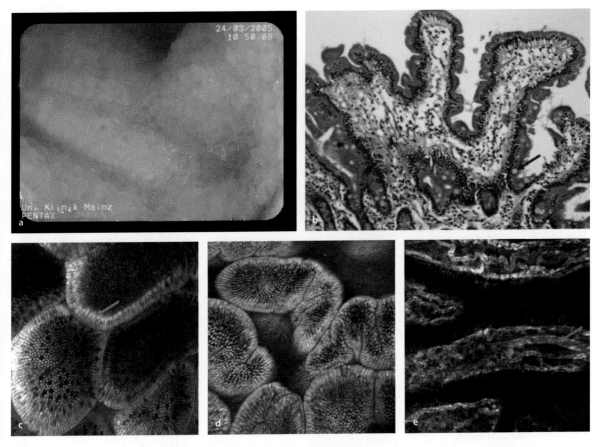

Fig. 6.9a–e. Small bowel architecture: endoscopy, endomicroscopy and histology. **a** White-light endoscopy of the terminal ileum: Multiple villi can be seen. **b** Conventional histology of small bowel architecture shows cellular detail with nuclei (*orange arrow*) of epithelial cells and mucin within epithelial cells defining goblet cells. **c** Acriflavine staining leads to visualisation of nuclei (*orange arrow*) and goblet cells (*blue arrow*). In endomicroscopy mucin within cells is displayed dark, whereas in conventional histology goblet cells are displayed very bright due to formalin fixation of specimens. **d** Overview of microscopic architecture of villi seen with acriflavine-aided endomicroscopy. **e** Endomicroscopy especially highlights capillaries. Here, the capillary network within the lamina propria within single villi is readily visible. Even single erythrocytes within the capillaries can be seen

the mucosa consists of two main cell types, namely the absorptive columnar cells and the mucus-secreting goblet cells. The columnar cells are the most abundant and are responsible for ionic regulation and water resorption. The goblet cells secrete mucus required for lubrication and are more abundant in the base of the glands. The number of cells within the lamina propria decreases from the proximal colon to the rectum. Normally, lymphocytes and plasma cells are found in the colon, but no neutrophilic granulocytes are present. Pathological changes in the colon may involve the mucosa, as in chronic inflammatory bowel disease, the number and kind of cells within the tunica propria, and the number and kind of cells within the lumen of crypts, and may involve the subepithelial layer as well, as in collagenous colitis.

6.3.8 Endomicroscopic Imaging of Colonic Mucosa

The mucosal surface of the colon is composed of thousands of crypts orientated as straight tubular structures

6

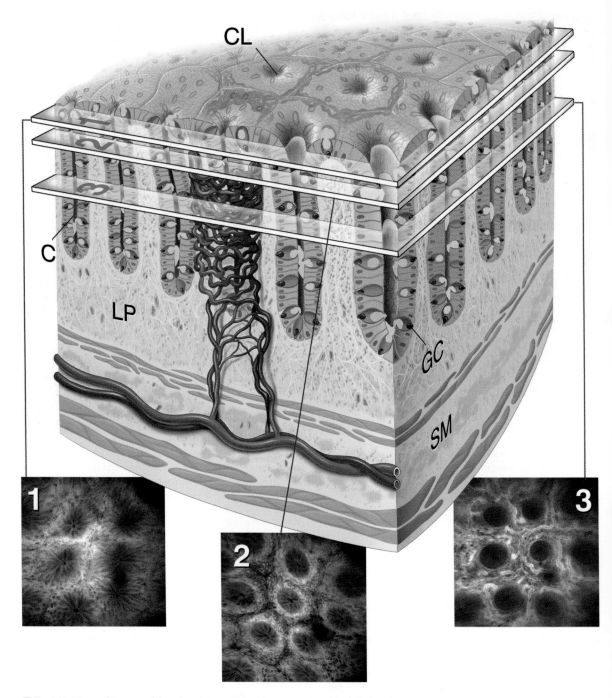

◧ **Fig. 6.10.** Microarchitecture of the colon. *C* Crypt, *LP* lamina propria, *GC* goblet cell, *SM* submucosa

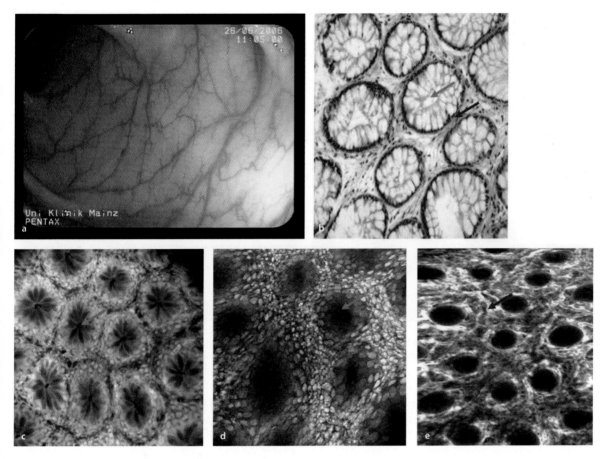

Fig. 6.11a–e. Colonic architecture: endoscopy, endomicroscopy and histology. **a** Macroscopic view of the sigmoid colon. The regular vasculature is visible. **b** Conventional histology shows the luminal openings of crypts (*arrow*). The crypts contain epithelial cells and goblet cells. The nuclei within the epithelial cells are displayed as dark purple areas using classical H&E staining. **c** Endomicroscopy with fluorescein shows the regular architecture of crypts in horizon- tal section. The lumen (*arrow*) and cells and the intercryptal epithelial cells can be seen. **d** Acriflavine highlights cell membranes and nuclei. However, the overall architecture of crypts is also clearly visible (*arrow* within the lumen of a single crypt). **e** The capillaries within the lamina propria can be best visualised in the middle portion of the mucosal layer. Here, fluorescein leads to a bright contrast of capillaries (*blue arrow*)

extending down to the muscularis mucosae (Figs. 6.10, 6.9). The intravenous administration of fluorescein (5– 10ml of a 10% solution) results in strong staining of the surface epithelium and the deeper layers of the lamina propria. When imaged en face using confocal endomi- croscopy, the luminal openings of the crypts are observed as black holes projecting onto the surface and the epithe- lial cell types (i.e. columnar cells and goblet cells) can be clearly distinguished (image 1 of Fig. 6.10). Just below the surface, the mouth of the crypt slopes gently like a funnel and the epithelial cells types are radially orientated within the crypt lumen. The BM forms a boundary between the

epithelium and the lamina propria (image 2 of Fig. 6.10). The capillaries of the colonic mucosa are contained within the lamina propria and form a honeycomb-like network around each crypt (image 3 of Fig. 6.10).

6.4 Lymphoid Tissue

In general, lymphoid tissue in the gastrointestinal tract is known as mucosa-associated lymphatic tissue (MALT) or gut-associated lymphatic tissue (GALT). Lymphoid nod- ules are almost exclusively confined to the terminal ileum,

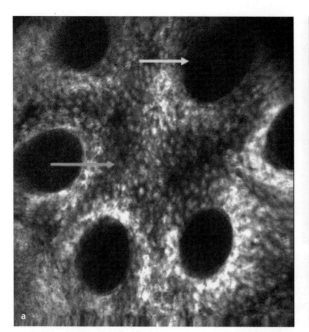
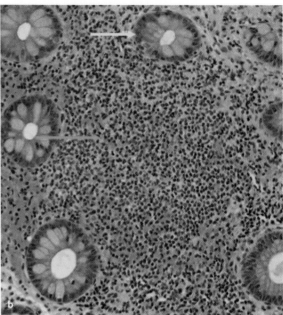

■ Fig. 6.12a,b. Lymph follicle in the colon. **a** Endomicroscopy leads to identification of crypts (*yellow arrow*) and roundish lymphocytes (*green arrow*) within the lamina propria. **b** Same features are seen in conventional histology after targeted biopsies

while other parts of the gastrointestinal tract contain more diffusely arranged lymphocytes and other immune cells. Lymphoid follicles in otherwise healthy mucosa may be a sign of prior infection. If numerous lymphoid follicles are present during routine endoscopy, then an underlying condition such as chronic infections or follicular lymphoma needs to be excluded.

Single lymphatic aggregates can be found in the oesophagus, gastric corpus, small intestine, and large intestine without any further pathological meaning (■ Fig. 6.12). The lymphoid tissue communicates with the epithelial cells to ensure host defences against luminal antigens. The number of these lymphoid cells increases with age and infection.

Most intraepithelial lymphocytes belong to the suppressor T-cell group and can be identified immunohistochemically with CD8 antibodies. Dendritic cytoplasmic protrusions ensure tight contact with adjacent epithelial cells. Normally, plasma cells are not found in the epithelium, but they are interepithelial within the tunica propria between the glands.

Acquired lymphoid tissue in the gut can give rise to lymphoma, such as marginal cell lymphoma, which is found in the stomach during chronic *Helicobacter pylori* infection. In the stomach typical lymphoepithelial destruction of glands is a histological sign of infiltration by a low-grade MALT lymphoma. Such glandular destruction is rarely found in the lower gastrointestinal tract in cases of colonic lymphoma. Mucosal plasma cells produce IgA and IgM antibody dimers and pentamers that migrate to the crypt membrane of the small and large bowel and occasionally to the stomach. The epithelium produces a secretory component to which the antibodies bind; they are then secreted together through endocytic vesicles into the lumen.

Different types of cells can be observed endomicroscopically within the lamina propria. Lymphocytes can be identified due to their characteristic oval shape and size. However, due to the lack of nuclei staining when intravenous fluorescein is used, white blood cells are difficult to differentiate.

6.5   Innervation

The gastrointestinal innervation is partially independent from the brain and can provide direct reflex activity. The whole gut is innervated by autonomic motor and sensory neurons. At the moment the neural »gut-brain axis« is one of the hottest topics in the scientific literature, although the implications of this axis are not yet clear. Diseases such as irritable bowel syndrome are believed to derive from a dysregulation of such an axis or of the peripheral autonomic regulation by the gastrointestinal plexus. Within the neural system sensory neurons detect the volume, composition, fluidity and temperature of food and other luminal contents. On exposure to food and luminal content, local neurotransmitters are released immediately within the gastrointestinal interneural circuits of the submucosal ganglia. These neurotransmitters can react with the appropriate receptors or with other neurons. The activation of motor neurons is triggered by the release of certain neurotransmitters. These nerves follow the blood vessels to ensure innervation of the vessel musculature and also run parallel to the vessels and terminate in the enteric ganglia or as free nerve endings.

Free nerve endings are believed to be responsible for pain reception, especially in the oesophagus. These nerve endings are not easy to detect with routine histological methods and require immunohistochemical or sliver impregnation techniques. In endomicroscopy, nerves cannot be identified with the currently available contrast agents.

6.6   Endocrine Cells

Supporting the autonomic nervous system of the gastrointestinal tract are endocrine cells; these can be found throughout the GI tract including the pancreas. They can occur as single cells or in clusters. Morphologically, these cells are easily identified through their typical appearance and their reaction to silver impregnation (argentaffinic cells) and to potassium dichromate (enterochromaffin cells). Those reacting only to silver in conjunction with an additional reducing component are called argyrophilic. At least 12 different types of endocrine-paracrine cells have been recognised. However, not all of the 20 known gastrointestinal hormones can be localised to specific cell types so far. Future functional intravital methods with endomicroscopy could eventually provide this missing information using specific contrast agents. Currently, endomicroscopy is not able to identify enterochromaffin cells.

Neuroendocrine tumours can be composed of hormonally active or inactive cells. The biological behaviour of these tumours is dependent on tumour size, the presence or absence of vessel penetration, and site. For example, neuroendocrine tumours of the terminal ileum often show malignant behaviour, while neuroendocrine tumours of the stomach, particularly in autoimmune gastritis, frequently show a favourable clinical course.

6.7   Vasculature

The blood supply and lymphatic system of the gastrointestinal tract are determined by vessels entering from the surrounding tissue. The blood vessels with the largest diameter can be found in the submucosal layer, sending small arterioles and capillaries into the mucosa and the tissue below the submucosal layer. In the muscularis, the vessels are arranged in a parallel manner to avoid loss of blood flow during muscle contraction. In the mucosal layer, such as in the oesophageal mucosa, irregular capillary loops may be present, where small veins anastomose with the arterial system in the submucosal layer.

Lymphatic vessels are very small in the mucosal layer and somewhat difficult to identify. In chronic inflammatory bowel conditions such as Crohn's disease, the lymphatic vessels in the mucosa become visible due to the surrounding scarring and the subsequent dilatation of these vessels. In normal mucosa, most of the lymphatic vessels are collapsed and thus not readily identifiable.

Endomicroscopy with fluorescein can be ideally used for identifying vessels in the mucosa. Capillaries are brightly highlighted and the different blood cells can be observed. Changes in vessel architecture can be used to diagnose inflammation and neoplasia. Fluorescein allows ready identification of the capillary network right after the i.v. injection, whereas acriflavine leads to a delayed staining of the capillaries after it has been absorbed in the vessels. Afterwards, even endothelial cells can be identified.

6.8   Conclusion

In conclusion, conventional histology and endomicroscopy are supplementary tools and show different image characteristics. Conventional histology provides a static view of microscopic changes of the mucosal layer and, after deep biopsies, even from the submucosal layer. Biopsy specimens have to be prepared (fixation and staining) before a microscopic tissue analysis can be made. Several dyes are available, highlighting different cells or components within the tissue specimen.

Knowledge of the microarchitecture of the mucosa is mandatory before starting endomicroscopy, because the identification of regular architecture will subsequently avoid regular mucosal biopsy. Endomicroscopy provides in vivo horizontal optical sections of the mucosal layer. An optical biopsy consists of different images at different depth levels within a defined mucosal area. Thus, the examiner has to put the information from different images together to form a final conclusion. Endomicroscopic imaging allows a rapid evaluation even from larger areas of the mucosa. However, endomicroscopy is always the combination of white-light endoscopy (macroscopy), with or without auxiliary techniques defining an area of interest, and subsequent microscopic analysis with the confocal device. The advantage of endomicroscopy is the immediate »online« and functional analysis of the mucosal layer. The endoscopist or endomicroscopist is challenged to find an in vivo diagnosis leading to targeted biopsy or endoscopic therapy.

References

1   Fazzini E, Weber D, Waldo E (1972) A manual for surgical pathologists. Thomas, Springfield
2   Underwood JCE (1981) Introduction to biopsy interpretation and surgical pathology. Springer, Berlin Heidelberg New York
3   Bonk U (1983) Biopsie und Operationspräparat. Kompendium für Ärzte und Studenten. Karger, Basel
4   Böck P (ed) (1989) Romeis mikroskopische Technik, 17th edn. Urban & Schwarzenberg, Munich
5   Fenoglio-Preiser CM, Lantz PE, Listrom MB, Davis M, Rilke FO (1989) Gastrointestinal pathology. Raven, New York
6   Atay Z, Topalides T (1994) Cytodiagnostik der serösen Höhlen. In: Atay Z, Topalides T (eds) Atlas und Lehrbuch. Pabst Verlag, Berlin
7   Sternberg SS, Antonioli DA, Carter D, Mills SE, Oberman HA (1994) Diagnostic surgical pathology, 2nd edn. Raven, Hagerstown
8   Rosai J (ed) (1996) Ackerman's surgical pathology, 8th edn. Mosby, St.Louis
9   Remmele W (ed) (1999) Pathologie 1, 2nd edn. Springer, Berlin Heidelberg New York Tokyo, pp 25-46
10 Ross MH, Pawlina W, Kaye GI (2003) Histology: a text and atlas. Lippincott Williams & Wilkins, Philadelphia Baltimore
11 Flenker H (2004) Taschenatlas der gynäkologischen Zytologie. IDWerk Bremerhaven
12 Standring S (ed) (2004) Gray's anatomy. Churchill Livingstone, Edinburgh

Endomicroscopy of GI Disorders

Key concepts:
- Endomicroscopy allows in vivo imaging of Barrett's esophagus, HP-induced gastritis and gastric cancer.
- In the small bowel, endomicroscopy permits analysis of pathologic changes in celiac disease and MALT lymphoma.
- Endomicroscopy can be used in patients with ulcerative colitis and microscopic colitis to target biopsies.

Endomicroscopy can be used to observe living cells during ongoing endoscopy. A multitude of changes can be identified by the endomicroscopist. Thus, a thorough knowledge about mucosal pathology is mandatory to obtain a reliable online diagnosis.

The main goal of endomicroscopy is to identify mucosal areas suspicious for neoplasia or other changes, leading immediately to targeted biopsy or endoscopic therapy. This chapter gives an overview of the currently available endomicroscopic classifications and describes several common diseases of the GI tract. Note that close interaction with the pathologist is needed to achieve a complete diagnosis and to further expand the diagnostic possibilities of endomicroscopy.

7.1 Endomicroscopy in Early Oesophageal Squamous Cell Neoplasias

Oliver Pech, Christian Ell

The incidence of squamous cell cancer of the oesophagus has decreased in Western countries over the past few years, it being 4–16/100 000 depending on geographical location, with higher rates in Asia [1]. When oesophageal cancer is limited to the mucosa, endoscopic therapy using endoscopic resection (ER) or photodynamic therapy (PDT) can be performed with curative intent [1–4]. ER has been established as a standard treatment for patients with early squamous cell neoplasia during the past several years. Several reports, first from Asia but recently from Western countries, have revealed promising results, especially when cancerous tissue is limited to the mucosa (m1–m3) [4, 5]. These patients with limited disease have a very low risk for lymph node metastasis and can be cured by endoscopic therapy. In contrast, in cases of submucosal invasion, the rate of lymph node malignancy rises to 50% and the outcome after ER is poor [4, 6].

The diagnosis of discrete squamous cell neoplasia in the oesophagus can be facilitated by chromoendoscopy with Lugol's iodine solution. Iodine stains glycogen on the surface of the oesophageal squamous epithelium, resulting in a brownish appearance of normal tissue. Glycogen is not expressed on the surface of neoplastic mucosa and these areas remain unstained. Typically, biopsies are taken from these unstained areas and neoplasia must be confirmed by a pathologist, with definitive endoscopic therapy subsequently carried out some days later. Confocal laser endomicroscopy (CLE) enables the endoscopist to acquire histological images in vivo and to proceed immediately to ER of the lesion if malignancy is confirmed. In addition, endoscopic ultrasound might be added to rule out malignant infiltration or determine its depth.

Endomicroscopic images of normal squamous cell epithelium show regular architecture of the cells and capillaries (◘ Fig. 7.1a,b). Neoplastic epithelium appears different, and is characterised by irregular cell architecture, leakage of fluorescein out of the capillaries into the surrounding tissue; elongation and irregular twisting of the capillaries can also be observed (◘ Fig. 7.2a–d) [7]. The

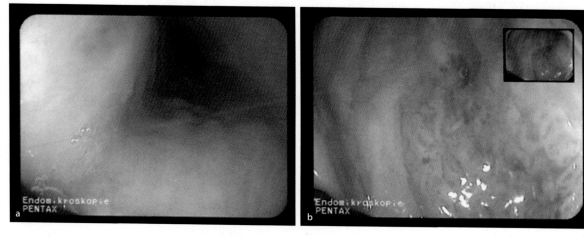

◘ **Fig. 7.1a,b.** Squamous cell cancer of the oesophagus. **a** Normal squamous epithelium is visible in the upper third of the oesophagus. **b** An irregular, flat mucosal lesion can be identified in the middle third of the oesophagus

◘ **Fig. 7.2a–d.** Endomicroscopy and histology of normal squamous epithelium and oesophageal cancer. **a** The bright bands represent intrapapillary capillaries, which are highlighted due to fluorescein administration. The dye uptake within epithelial cells is weak in normal epithelium. Thus, single cells can hardly be differentiated. In addition, fluorescein does not display nuclei due to pharmacokinetic properties. **b** Conventional histology with H&E staining provides information about nuclei and capillaries. Regular shape and size of nuclei can be seen, with increased cellularity around the capillaries. **c** Highly irregular cell architecture is visible and leakage of fluoresecein is seen as very bright irregular spots within the tissue; this is highly suspicious for the presence of neoplasia. **d** Histology confirms the presence of a moderate differentiated squamous cell cancer

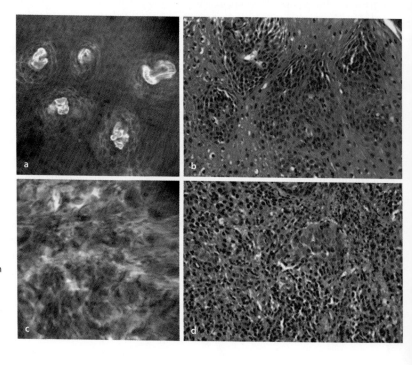

endomicroscopic images of squamous cell oesophageal cancer correspond well with conventional histology, and clinical decision-making can usually rely on the diagnosis made in vivo.

However, in cases where in vivo histology is uncertain, endoscopists should still rely on mucosal biopsy and wait for the pathological diagnosis before deciding whether further diagnostic or therapeutic procedures are needed.

References

1. Messmann H (2001) Squamous cell cancer of the oesophagus. Best Pract Res Clin Gastroenterol 15:249–265
2. Takeshita K, Tani M, Inoue H, et al (1997) Endoscopic treatment of early esophageal or gastric cancer. Gut 40:123–127
3. Makuuchi H (1996) Endoscopic mucosal resection for early esophageal cancer: indication and techniques. Dig Endosc 8:175–179
4. Pech O, Gossner L, May A, Vieth M, Stolte M, Ell C (2004) Endoscopic resection of superficial esophageal squamous-cell carcinomas: Western experience. Am J Gastroenterol 99:1226–1232
5. Pech O, May A, Gossner L, Rabenstein T, Manner H, Huijsmans J, Vieth M, Stolte M, Berres M, Ell C (2007) Curative endoscopic therapy in patients with early esophageal squamous cell carcinoma and high grade intraepithelial neoplasia. Endoscopy (in press)
6. Stein HJ, Feith M, Bruecher BL, Naehrig J, Sarbia M, Siewert JR (2005) Early esophageal cancer: pattern of lymphatic spread and prognostic factors for long-term survival after surgical resection. Ann Surg 242:566–573
7. Deinert K, Kiesslich R, Vieth M, Neurath MF, Neuhaus H (2007) In-vivo microvascular imaging of early squamous-cell cancer of the oesophagus by confocal laser endomicroscopy. Endoscopy (in press)

7.2 Barrett's Oesophagus

Ralf Kiesslich, Kerry Dunbar, Markus F. Neurath

Barrett's oesophagus is known to be a premalignant condition in patients with gastroesophageal reflux disease, and most adenocarcinomas of the distal oesophagus have been shown to arise in Barrett's tissue. Barrett's oesophagus is defined histologically by the presence of specialised columnar epithelium (SCE) with goblet cells. The columnar-lined lower oesophagus can be identified during standard upper endoscopy. SCE is often present in a patchy mosaic contribution within columnar-lined lower oesophagus and can be overlooked by random biopsies, resulting in biopsies of the cardia or gastric type of mucosa without goblet cells. However, it has been suggested that four-quadrant step biopsies within the columnar-lined lower oesophagus should serve as the gold standard for diagnosing Barrett's epithelium and Barrett's-associated neoplastic changes.

Endomicroscopy makes it possible to identify columnar-lined lower oesophagus macroscopically and identify goblet cells microscopically in the distal oesophagus, allowing an immediate and reliable diagnosis of Barrett's oesophagus. In the first endomicroscopic study about Barrett's oesophagus with 63 patients, different types of epithelial cells were distinguishable, and cellular and vascular changes were detected using fluorescein-guided endomicroscopy [1]. A classification of confocal images for the diagnosis of Barrett's epithelium and Barrett's-associated neoplasias was developed on the basis of a comparison of the in vivo and conventional ex vivo histology (◘ Table 7.1). The classification distinguishes between three types of epithelium (gastric epithelium; Barrett's epithelium without neoplastic changes; and Barrett's epithelium with neoplastic changes).

Confocal imaging of the normal squamous epithelium of the oesophagus demonstrated squamous cells at high resolution, showing capillaries (filled with red blood cells) within single papillae (◘ Fig. 7.1b). It also became obvious that the number of papillae appears to increase after damage to the epithelium (e.g. in erosive oesophagitis). It is possible to diagnose dilated intercellular spaces, which can be seen in patients with oesophageal damage. Analysis of the Z-line showed the clear border between squamous and columnar-lined epithelium. Goblet cells, which are pathognomonic for Barrett's epithelium, are easily identified. The mucin (MUC2) in goblet cells appears as dark spots within single cells of CLE (◘ Fig. 7.3). The typical shape of Barrett's epithelium is villous with the presence of a brush border, differing from the cardiac epithelium. High-grade intraepithelial neoplasias or early cancers can be recognised by a distinct cell type in endomicroscopy. The highly irregular and polygonal cells have a rather black appearance, with irregular borders (◘ Fig. 7.4). In addition, an irregular epithelial cell layer with typical black cells and loss of a regular basal border is found, indicating high-grade intraepithelial neoplasia. The brightness of the lamina propria becomes heterogeneous due to the mixed vasculature of neoangiogenesis and leakage phenomena (◘ Fig. 7.4).

In the first study dealing with endomicroscopy in patients with Barrett's oesophagus [1], 156 areas and 3012

▫ Table 7.1. Endomicroscopic classification of Barrett's oesophagus

Confocal diagnosis	Vessel architecture	Crypt architecture
Gastric-type epithelium	Capillaries with a regular shape only visible in the deeper parts of the mucosal layer	Regular columnar-lined epithelium with round glandular openings and typical cobblestone appearance
Barrett's epithelium	Subepithelial capillaries with a regular shape underneath columnar-lined epithelium visible in the upper and deeper parts af the mucosal layer	Columnar-lined epithelium with intermittent dark mucin in goblet cells in the upper parts of the mucosal layer. In the deeper parts, villous, dark, regular cylindrical Barrett's epithelial cells are present
Neoplasia	Irregular capillaries visible in the uper and deeper parts of the Mucosal layer. Leakage of vessels leads to a heterogeneous and brighter signal intensity within the lamina propria	Black cells with irregular apical and distal borders and shapes, with strong dark contrast against the surrounding tissue

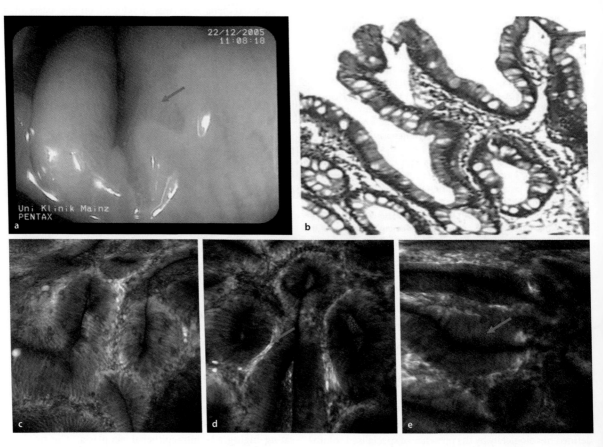

▫ Fig. 7.3a–e. Endomicroscopy of non-dysplastic Barrett's oesophagus. **a** White-light endoscopy of the distal oesophagus. Columnar-lined lower oesophagus is present with a single, short, reddish tongue visible. **b** Histology of non-dysplastic Barrett's epithelium. The goblet cells (*arrow*) within columnar epithelium are pathognomonic for Barrett's epithelium. **c** Endomicroscopy with fluorescein shows cylindrical epithelial cells within the distal oesophagus, defining metaplasia. Goblet cells within columnar epithelium are present and Barrett's epithelium can be diagnosed. **d** Small-calibre capillaries lie directly beneath the basement membrane. **e** In deeper parts of the epithelium the typical arrangement of Barrett's glands is visible (*arrow*). A brush border is located at the apical site of the epithelial cells

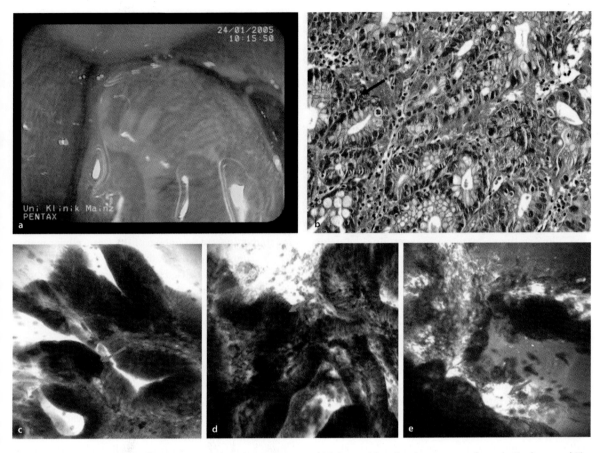

Fig. 7.4a–e. Endomicroscopy of Barrett's-associated neoplasia. **a** A subtle lesion with shallow protrusion and central depression is visible within known Barrett's oesophagus. **b** Mucosal biopsy showing highly irregular glands and nuclei (*arrow*) with increase of vasculature. **c** Endomicroscopy with fluorescein displays the abrupt change of architecture within columnar-lined lower oesophagus, which is suspicious for the presence of neoplastic changes. **d** The overall architecture becomes highly irregular at the central part of the lesion, with loss of polarity of malignant cells at the epithelial level (*arrow*)and within the lamina propria. **e** The capillaries show strong leakage with pooling of fluorescein within the lamina propria, indicating neoangiogenesis

images were reassessed in accordance with the newly developed confocal Barrett's classification and compared with the targeted biopsies (411 biopsies). The comparison showed that Barrett's oesophagus could be predicted based on the identification of goblet cells with the help of confocal endomicroscopy with a sensitivity of 98.1% and a specificity of 94.1% (accuracy 96.8%; positive predictive value 97.2%; negative predictive value 96.0%). Moreover, Barrett's-associated neoplastic changes could be predicted based on irregular black cells with a sensitivity of 92.9% and a specificity of 98.4%, (accuracy 97.4%; positive predictive value 92.9%; negative predictive value 98.4%).

Reference

1. Kiesslich R, Gossner L, Dahlmann A et al (2006) In vivo histology of Barrett's oesophagus and associated neoplasias by confocal laser endomicroscopy. Clin Gastroenterol Hepatol 8:979–987

7.3   Endomicroscopy of Gastritis and Gastric Cancer

Katja Wirths, Horst Neuhaus

Endoscopy and histopathology are approaching each other more and more. Sophisticated techniques such as chromoendoscopy and enhanced magnification give detailed information about the gastrointestinal surface structure. Several studies have demonstrated the value of these techniques, with regard to the stomach, particularly for differentiation between neoplastic and non-neoplastic changes. Chromoendoscopy is used to highlight the pit pattern structure of the mucosal surface, allowing the endoscopist to determine the nature of gastric lesions from indirect criteria. Magnification endoscopy is able to visualise surface structures with increased detail due to magnification factors of 80–150. However, neither of these techniques is able to look below the mucosal surface. Confocal laser endomicroscopy (CLE) enables a microscopic tissue analysis in vivo during ongoing endoscopy. The magnification factor in endomicroscopy is about $1000 \times$ and permits the analysis of tissue pattern and microvascular architecture. For an adequate interpretation of the confocal images a knowledge of histopathology and of the endomicroscopic appearance of normal tissue is essential, especially where non-neoplastic versus neoplastic changes are concerned.

7.3.1   Normal Gastric Microarchitecture

Due to the limited laser penetration depth of about 250 μm, endomicroscopy images epithelial cells and most parts of the lamina propria. The technique allows the investigation of mucosal vessels as well as tissue architecture. Capillaries surround each crypt and communicate with each other through a visible vascular network. Collecting venules are occasionally seen in the mucosa of the gastric body. Larger vessels such as arterioles are localised in the submucosal layer and therefore can not be visualised with CLE [1].

Mucosal capillaries show a characteristic appearance depending on their topographic location. In the body of the stomach, capillaries form a »honeycomb« network. In the deeper mucosal parts of the antrum the typical architecture of the capillaries shows spiral or coil-shaped struc-

tures forming a capillary network. These observations are consistent with mucosal surface findings identified by magnification endoscopy (◘ Fig. 7.5a, b) [2].

The pit architecture also varies depending on the anatomical site. The pits in the body of the stomach are usually regular with roundish luminal openings. In the fundus, round luminal openings of the gastric glands represent the endomicroscopic equivalent of the type I pit pattern classification in magnification endoscopy established by Guelrud [3]. The crypts of the antrum are longer or rigid [4]. On the surface, regular antral mucosa forms a cobblestone pattern (◘ Fig. 7.5).

The columnar cells are visualised as regularly shaped and sized cells with small, bright intercellular spaces due to the fluorescein uptake of the extracellular matrix [5]. In contrast to histopathological examination, the nuclei are not visualised when fluorescein sodium is used. By combining these characteristic vascular, cell and tissue features, examiners are able to determine the topographic anatomy without being aware of the region examined [4].

7.3.2   Gastritis

Histopathologically, gastritis is defined by various stages of inflammatory change. These include infiltration of the lamina propria by inflammatory cells and alteration and defects of the mucosal surface such as erosions. Diagnosis of gastritis by endomicroscopy with fluorescein sodium relies mainly on three factors: increased cellularity in the lamina propria, glands without neoplastic changes and regular microvascular arrangement. Due to the fact that fluorescein does not stain the nuclei themselves, differentiation of different types of white blood cells is not yet possible. The endomicroscopic grading of the inflammatory changes has also not yet been defined. Typical gastritis-related changes visualised during endomicroscopy include an increase of cells in the lamina propria. The architecture of the gastric glands is maintained. In cases of chronic erosive changes or ulcers when the glands have vanished, the connective tissue may be rich in new capillaries or may show necrosis, depending on the phase of the healing process. Especially in *Helicobacter pylori*-positive acute gastritis, the vascularity may be increased [6]. Still, the margins of the remaining gastric epithelium demonstrate a non-neoplastic glandular architecture. The intensity of tissue fluorescence is probably dependent on

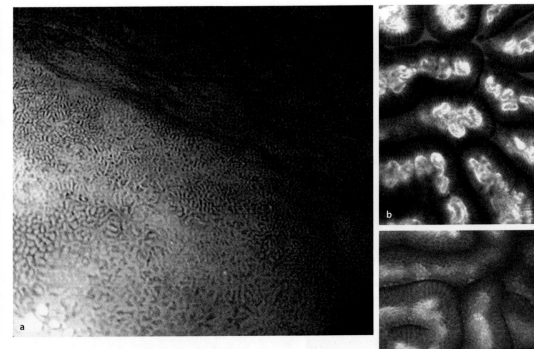

☐ Fig. 7.5a–c. Macroscopic and microscopic appearance of gastric mucosa. **a** Endoscopic aspect of regular gastric mucosa visualised by narrow band imaging (NBI) technique. The regularly arranged mucosal microvessel architecture of the antrum is highlighted by NBI. **b** Corresponding endomicroscopic aspect of regular antral mucosa. Mucosal microvessels are bright due to the uptake of florescein sodium. In the gastric antrum, microvessels build a regular coil-shaped capillary network. **c** Cobblestone appearance of the superficial gastric mucosa visualised by CLE with fluorescein sodium

the amount of stroma present. Bhunchet and co-workers demonstrated a higher fluorescence in diseases with increased stroma and fewer glands in comparison to the surrounding tissue [7].

7.3.3 Intestinal Metaplasia

Intestinal metaplasia in the stomach is assumed to be at least a precancerous marker of gastric malignancy. It is commonly detected in reactive chemical gastritis in the antrum and in chronic atrophic gastritis found in the gastric corpus. The histopathological criterion of intestinal metaplasia is the presence of goblet cells. Usually, these mucin-filled cells are found in the epithelial layer of the colon and small intestine but not in the normal stomach. The occurrence of goblet cells in

the columnar epithelium of the stomach is pathognomonic for intestinal metaplasia. Endomicroscopically, goblet cells appear as homogeneous dark spots almost filling a complete epithelial columnar cell and can be readily identified (☐ Figs. 7.6a,b, ☐ Fig. 7.7). Thus, they are detected with low interobserver variability [8] and confirm the assumption of chronic atrophic gastritis if detected in the corpus.

7.3.4 *Helicobacter pylori*-positive Gastritis

The detection of *Helicobacter pylori* (HP) colonisation has several diagnostic and therapeutic implications, since eradication reduces the risk of ulcer recurrence. Additionally, eradication is first-line treatment for stage-I gastric MALT lymphomas. Kiesslich et al. were able to show that

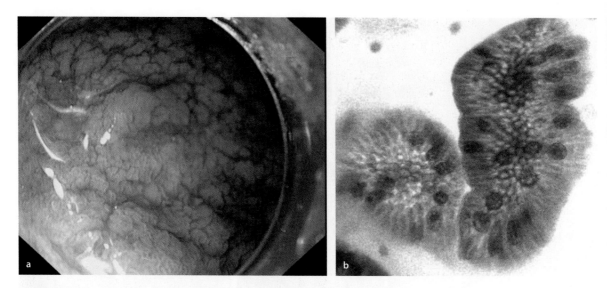

▣ Fig. 7.6a,b. Atrophic gastritis. **a** Endoscopic aspect of chronic atrophic gastritis with intestinal metaplasia after topical application of indigo carmine. **b** Superficial endomicroscopic aspect of **a**, showing dark round dots in some of the epithelial cells representing mucin-filled goblet cells

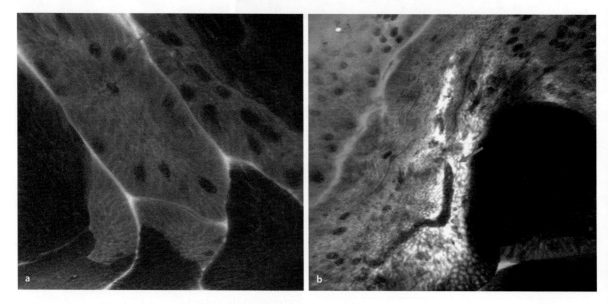

▣ Fig. 7.7a,b. Atrophic gastritis and gastric cancer. **a** Intestinal metaplasia within the stomach is visible due to the presence of goblet cells (*arrow*). **b** Intestinal metaplasia is in transition to gastric cancer (*dark cells*). Within the transition zone an altered vessel is visible (*arrow*) which ends abruptly, and the contrast agent fluorescein is flows into the lamina propria, leading to bright contrast

acriflavine, a topical fluorescent dye, is able to label HP. Acriflavine appears to be actively taken up by the HP bacteria. Following endoscopic laser stimulation, the bacteria are easily detected due to their characteristic morphology [9] (▣ Fig. 7.8). The endomicroscopic detection was independent of the density or distribution of HP bacteria and even individual bacteria could be identified. This enables a targeted biopsy and may therefore decrease the rate of false-negative diagnoses by eliminating non-representative conventional biopsies.

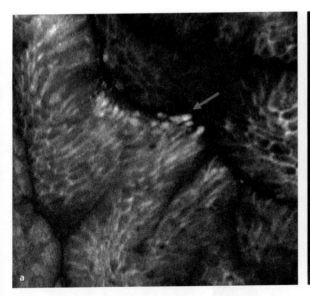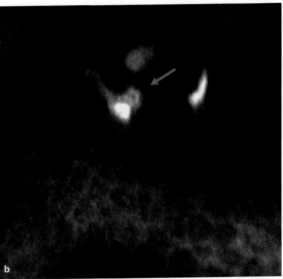

Fig. 7.8a,b. *Helicobacter pylori*-associated gastritis. **a** Bright germs can be identified on the surface of gastric epithelium (*arrow*) following fluorescein injection and topical acriflavine application. Acriflavine is accumulated in *H. pylori* and leads to bright contrast of bacteria. **b** Single germs can be highlighted even more using acriflavine alone. The typical shape of *H. pylori* can be observed at high contrast

7.3.5 Early Gastric Cancer

Early detection of gastric neoplasia is important, since early gastric cancer (EGC) confined to the mucosal layer and focal invasion into the submucosal layer is curable by local endoscopic therapy [10, 11]. The endoscopic detection of EGC is challenging, as these lesions usually are non-polypoid in contrast to colorectal lesions. Characteristic alterations suspicious for gastric neoplasia are changes in mucosal colour and surface structure. Chromoendoscopy and/or magnification endoscopy are used to detect and characterise these mucosal alterations. In the colonic mucosa, a pit pattern classification has been established demonstrating a correlation between histology and surface analysis [12]. A similar pit pattern classification for the stomach has not been established, probably due to the complexity of various mucosal patterns depending on the site examined. The most important goal with CLE in the stomach is to detect and biopsy suspicious lesions using optical-guided biopsies for histopathological confirmation.

Endomicroscopic-guided optical biopsies allow immediate microscopic analysis during ongoing endoscopy. Intra-individual comparison of regular and altered gastric mucosa facilitates the interpretation of the confocal images.

Yeoh was able to demonstrate a high accuracy in predicting the characteristic features of cancer in comparison to normal mucosa, chronic gastritis and intestinal metaplasia with a low interobserver variability [8]. Currently, of course, biopsies are still needed to confirm the endomicroscopic diagnosis. However, endomicroscopy can be used to guide biopsies to microscopically suspicious areas.

Characteristic neoplastic features of the gastric mucosa observed by CLE are changes in tissue and microvessel architecture as well as in cell morphology. The glands vary in size and shape with corresponding differences in luminal crypt openings (Figs. 7.9–7.11). The tissue pattern is disorganised or totally destroyed. The neoplastic columnar cells themselves are often dark and polygonal (Fig. 7.11). By directing the optical plane to the surface of the lesion, CLE may produce cytology-like microscopic images (Fig. 7.12b). Due to the properties of fluorescein sodium, nuclei are not stained. Acriflavine, a topical fluorescent stain, stains the nuclei and might be used for this purpose either alone or in conjunction with intravenous fluorescein sodium. The assessment of morphological differences between regular and neoplastic nuclei, especially with regard to size, offers another opportunity to diagnose gastric malignancies by CLE.

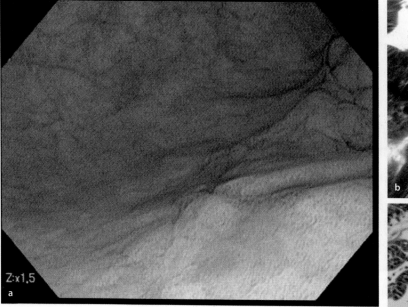

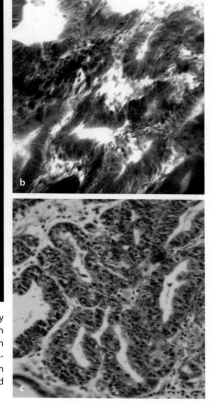

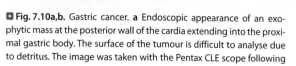

▣ **Fig. 7.9a–c.** Early gastric cancer. **a** Macroscopic aspect of a slightly elevated and centrally depressed lesion (type IIa+c of the Paris Classification) in the proximal antrum of the stomach seen with electronic zoom magnification. **b** Confocal laser endomicroscopy of the lesion shown in **a**. Irregular crypt openings and a thickening of the epithelial layer are obvious. **c** Histopathological slice of the lesion, which was removed by endoscopic submucosal dissection (ESD). The final histopathological diagnosis of the ESD specimen confirms a well-differentiated adenocarcinoma (UICC: pT1 (m-type), G1, pL0, pV0)

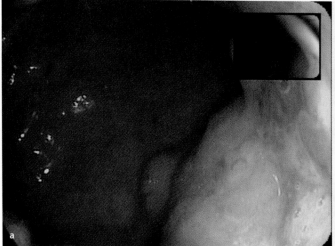

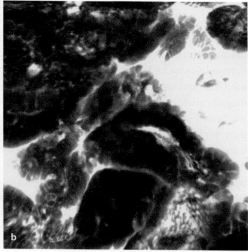

▣ **Fig. 7.10a,b.** Gastric cancer. **a** Endoscopic appearance of an exophytic mass at the posterior wall of the cardia extending into the proximal gastric body. The surface of the tumour is difficult to analyse due to detritus. The image was taken with the Pentax CLE scope following administration of fluorescein sodium. **b** CLE showing disorganised cell architecture with crowds of dark, neoplastic polygonal cells. Even irregular crypts are no longer visualised

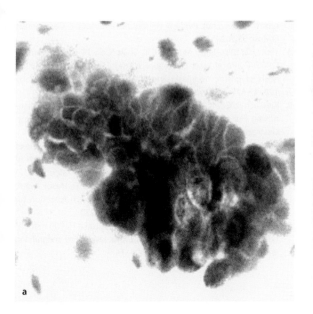
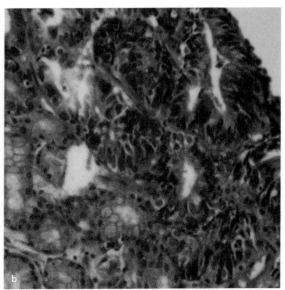

◨ **Fig. 7.11a,b.** Malignant cell analysis. **a** Superficial aspect of gastric neoplastic tissue with dark cells of irregular size and structure gathered together at the luminal surface. **b** Corresponding histopathology (biopsy specimen)

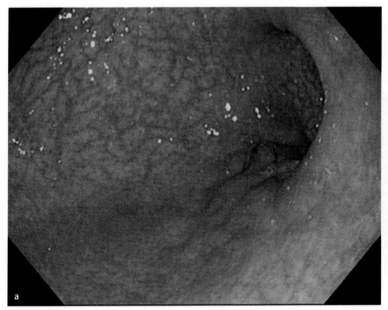
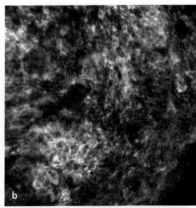
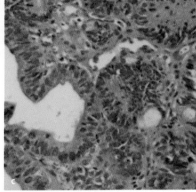

◨ **Fig. 7.12a–c.** Undifferentiated gastric cancer. **a** Type 2a+c neoplastic lesion in the gastric antrum, greater curve. **b** Corresponding CLE showing disorganised neoplastic tissue without any visible duct morphology. The characteristic gastric tissue with glands is completely replaced by the tumour. **c** Biopsy specimen of the lesion showing an undifferentiated adeno-carcinoma of the stomach. In some parts irregular glands are still visualised, whereas the majority of the tissue is completely destroyed

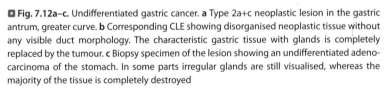

Vessels are usually located in the deeper part of the tumour and are often not visible by endomicroscopy. This phenomenon might also explain the »lack of vascularity« observed during magnification of EGC. Thus, the absence of a regular microvascular network contributes to the diagnosis of neoplasia by CLE as well.

Kitabatake et al. were able to show differences according to the grade of tumour differentiation by comparing CLE and histopathology of gastric cancer lesions. Disorganised neoplastic glands seem to be characteristic for a well-differentiated type of adenocarcinoma (🔲 Figs. 7.10 and 7.12). In contrast, in undifferentiated EGC the glands are not visualised. Instead, the neoplastic tissue consists of dark and polygonal neoplastic cell formations (🔲 Fig. 7.12). The accuracy for the diagnosis of gastric cancer by interpreting the CLE images in this trial was above 90% if a good image quality was provided [4].

In conclusion, confocal laser endomicroscopy in the stomach has the potential to diagnose intestinal metaplasia as a potential marker of chronic atrophic gastritis by imaging mucin-containing goblet cells, to predict HP colonisation even if the number of specimens is low, and to differentiate in vivo between benign and malignant lesions with a high accuracy.

References

1. Gannon B, Browning J, O'Brien P, Rogers P (1984) Mucosal microvascular architecture of the fundus and body of human stomach. Gastroenterology 86:866–875
2. Yao K (2004) Gastric microvascular architecture as visualized by magnifying endoscopy: body mucosa and antral mucosa without pathological change demonstrate two different patterns of micro vascular architecture. Gastrointest Endosc 59:596–597
3. Guelrud M, Ehrlich E (2004) Endoscopic classification of Barrett's oesophagus. Gastrointest Endosc 59:58–65
4. Kitabatake S, Niwa Y, Miyahara R, Ohashi A, Matsuura T, Iguchi Y, Shimoyama Y, Nagasaka Y, Maeda O, Ando T, Ohmiya N, Itoh A, Hirooka Y, Goto H (2006) Confocal endomicroscopy for the diagnosis of gastric cancer in vivo. Endoscopy 38:1110–1114
5. Polglase AL, McLaren WJ, Skinner SA, Kiesslich R, Neurath MF, Delaney PM (2005) A fluorescence confocal endomicroscope for in vivo microscopy of the upper- and lower-GI tract, Gastrointest Endosc 62:686–695
6. Tuccillo C, Cuomo A, Rocco A, Martinelli E, Staibano S, Mascolo M, Gravina AG, Nardone G, Ricci V, Ciardiello F, Del Vecchio Blanco C, Romano M (2005) Vascular endothelial growth factor and neoangiogenses in H. pylori gastritis in humans. J Pathol 207:277–284
7. Bhunchet E, Hatakawa H, Sakai Y, Shibata T (2002) Fluorescein electronic endoscopy: a novel method for detection of early stage gastric cancer not evident to routine endoscopy. Gastrointest Endosc 55:562–571
8. Yeoh KG, Salto-Tellez M, Khor CJL, Shah N, So JBY, Shen E, Ho KY (2005) Confocal Laser Endoscopy is useful for in-vivo rapid diagnosis of gastric neoplasia and pre-neoplasia. Gastroenterology 128 (4): A27-A27 Suppl.
9. Kiesslich R, Goetz M, Burg J, Stolte M, Siegel E, et al (2005) Diagnosing Helicobacter pylori in vivo by confocal laser endoscopy. Gastroenterology 128:2119–2123
10. Kojima T, Parra-Blanco A, Takahashi H, Fujita R (1998) Outcome of endoscopic mucosal resection for early gastric cancer: review of the Japanese literature. Gastrointest Endosc 48:550–555
11. Ono H, Gotoda T, Shirao K, Yamaguchi H, Saito D, Hosokawa K, Shimoda T, Yoshida S. (2001) Endoscopic mucosal resection for treatment of early gastric cancer. Gut 48:225–229
12. Kudo S, Tamura S, Nakajima T, Yamano H, Kusaka H, Watanabe H (1996) Diagnosis of colorectal tumorous lesions by magnifying endoscopy. Gastrointest Endosc 44:8–14

7.4 Endomicroscopy of Small Bowel Diseases: Coeliac Disease, Lymphoma

Arthur Hoffman, Ralf Kiesslich, Wolfgang Fischbach

The different components making up the complement of immune elements within the alimentary tract vary greatly. In contrast to the Waldeyer's ring region, the oesophagus and stomach are normally almost devoid of such immune apparatus, presumably because of the rapid transit of food and the chemically hostile environment for micro-organisms provided by salivary and gastric secretions. Only in pathological conditions, such as viral or fungal oesophageal infections, reflux oesophagitis or *Helicobacter* gastritis, does one encounter acquired mucosa-associated lymphoid tissue in these sites [1]. By contrast, the large and small bowel normally possess mucosa-associated lymphoid tissue (MALT), most visibly concentrated in the terminal ileum and appendix.

7.4.1 Coeliac Disease

In addition to surface cell analysis, subsurface imaging with endomicroscopy also unmasks changes in vessels, connective tissue and cellular architecture within the lamina propria during endoscopy. As a result, diseases normally diagnosed by conventional microscopic analysis only can now also be identified through in vivo histology [2]. Coeliac disease, also known as gluten-sensitive enteropathy or non-tropical or coeliac sprue, can be diagnosed by confocal endomicroscopy during examination of the small intestine. Gluten, a substance found in wheat, barley, and rye, reacts with the small bowel resulting in immunologically mediated inflammatory damage to the small-intestinal mucosa [3]. The endoscopic findings in coeliac disease include a loss or reduction of duodenal folds, scalloping of Kerckring's folds and a micronodular or mosaic duodenal mucosal pattern [3]. Despite the endoscopic findings, the diagnosis of coeliac disease is based on histological evaluation, being characterised by a loss of the villous structures and hyperplasia of the crypts. Furthermore, lymphocytes and plasma cells are found in the inflamed lamina propria and there is an increased density of intraepithelial lymphocytes, which can be described using the modified Marsh classification [5]. Confocal laser endomicroscopy (CLE) may be

an ideal tool for accurate diagnosis of coeliac disease during ongoing endoscopy, because it allows the identification of affected areas leading to targeted biopsies. The microscopic architecture of the small-intestinal mucosa can be displayed at subcellular resolution, enabling the identification of intraepithelial lymphocytes, epithelial and inflammatory changes including a decrease in epithelial villi (◘ Fig. 7.13). [Leong RWL, Koo JHK, Meredith CG, et al. Confocal laser endomicroscopy in the diagnosis of coeliac disease. Journal of Gastroenterology and Hepatology 21: A267-A267 Suppl. 4 Oct 2006.]

7.4.2 Gastrointestinal Lymphoma

The stomach and small intestine are the primary site of 20–30% of gastrointestinal lymphomas, or approximately

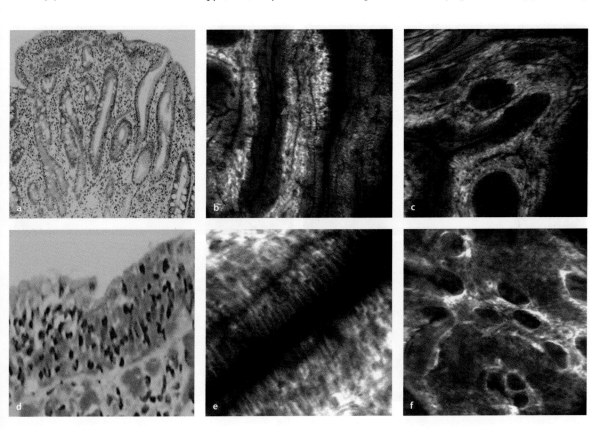

◘ **Fig. 7.13a–f.** Endomicroscopy in coeliac disease. **a** Coeliac disease is characterised by atrophy of villi (*arrow*) and an increase of lymphocytes in the lamina propria and especially within the epithelial layer. **b** Atrophy and reduction of villi length can be readily identified in vivo by performing endomicroscopy. **c** Villi are no longer visible in total atrophy, and the base of the crypts appears as roundish glands looking similar to colonic crypts. **d** Lymphocytes (*arrow*) can be identified within the epithelial layer in close observation. **e** Also endomicroscopy offers to identify intraepithelial lymphocytes (*arrow*). **f** Lymphocytes are also present in the lamina propria in further advanced disease

5% of peripheral non-Hodgkin's lymphomas (NHL) [4, 5]. Although substantial progress has been achieved in the diagnosis and treatment of intestinal lymphoma in recent years, the gastrointestinal lymphomas are still not well characterised, and standardised concepts for their clinical diagnosis and management are absent [6]. In almost all patients, the main tumour mass is located in the stomach or in the small bowel with a wide variety of macroscopic appearances [7]. An adequate histological classification is important for the management of intestinal lymphoma. Today the lymphomas are classified according to the Revised European-American Classification of Lymphoid Neoplasms. Further immunohistochemical and molecular tests are necessary for differentiation between B- and T-cell lymphomas [7].

7.4.3 Mantle-cell Lymphoma

Mantle-cell lymphoma has attained clear definition over the past decade, with both phenotypic and genetic criteria. Originally described by Lennert and co-workers in Kiel as 'centrocytic' lymphoma, and more vaguely in the USA as 'intermediately differentiated lymphocytic lymphoma', this neoplasm is now characterised as a spectrum of low-intermediate- to high-intermediate-grade B-cell tumours occurring predominantly in older men. There is a striking tendency for involvement of the GI tract, often as the spectacular phenomenon of lymphomatous polyposis [8] (◘ Fig. 7.14). This distinctive lymphoma grouping manifests CD5 co-expression with absence of CD23 in combination with cyclin D1 over-expression, on the basis

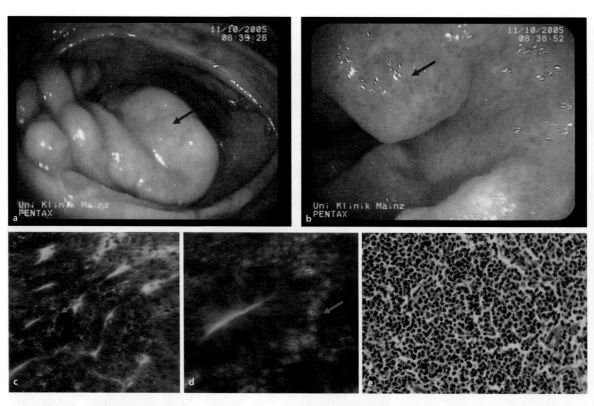

◘ **Fig. 7.14a–e.** Endomicroscopy of mantle cell lymphoma. **a** A tumorous lesion (*arrow*) is visible within the caecum, prolapsing out of the ileocaecal valve. **b** Protuberant lesions are also visible in the terminal ileum. **c** Endomicroscopy shows colonic architecture with an increased number of lymphocytes within the intercryptal space. **d** Further magnification shows the lining of bright lymphocytes in the lamina propria. Endomicroscopy cannot differentiate between different types of lymphoma. However, an increased number of lymphocytes with invasiveness into different portions of the mucosal layer can be readily identified. **e** Conventional histology of mantle cell lymphoma with H&E staining

of the Bcl-1 translocation, juxtaposing immunoglobulin encoding regions, most often of the heavy-chain region on chromosome 14, with the 'PRAD-1' oncogene region on chromosome 11 [9].

It is obvious that endomicroscopy cannot differentiate or readily identify malignant lymphoma. However, accumulation of lymphocytes can be identified due to the distinct shape of lymphocytes. The endoscopic changes can often be subtle. Here, endomicroscopy is able to recognise intraepithelial lymphocytes, leading to targeted biopsies, and subsequent nuclear staining for cyclin D1 is usually conclusive. It can be speculated that specific dyes might help in the future to characterise malignant lymphoma in vivo.

7.4.4 Proliferations of Acquired MALT

It is now established that certain external antigenic challenges, such as *Helicobacter*, can elicit the generation of acquired MALT, which resembles the normal lymphoid aggregates found in other gut locations, with follicles, mantle (dome) compartments, lamina propria elements, etc. However, for reasons not yet explained, the lympho-

mas arising from these acquired MALT tissues differ from those arising from lymphoid aggregates. In these acquired MALT tissues the cells primarily recognising the antigens are T cells, which induce proliferative B cells with autoimmune reactivity with local host tissue elements. Surprisingly, clinical remission of early MALT-type lymphomas can be achieved with antimicrobial therapy against *Helicobacter pylori* [10].

Low-grade B-cell lymphoma of extranodal marginal zone (MALT) type most often, but not invariably, arises in the stomach in relation to longstanding *Helicobacter* gastritis. Criteria for deciding the level of suspicion for lymphoma centre upon the degree of displacing atypical lymphoid infiltrate expanding the lamina propria [11]. Most experienced clinicians are comfortable with this. In many cases of low-grade MALT-type lymphoma isolated areas of an increased proportion of larger cells and increased mitotic activity are identified.

Endomicroscopy is able to identify intraepithelial lymphocytes and an increased amount of lymphocytes within the lamina propria. Macroscopic alterations in conjunction with the presence of a lymphocytic infiltration in the stomach might lead the endoscopist to the suspicion of the presence of MALT-lymphoma (□ Fig. 7.15). However,

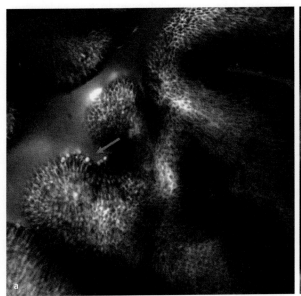
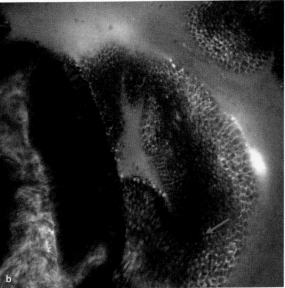

□ **Fig. 7.15a,b.** Endomicroscopy of MALT lymphoma of the stomach. **a** Distinct changes within the gastric mucosa. *Helicobacter pylori* are visible on top of an altered gastric gland (*arrow*). An increased cel-lularity of roundish cells is present surrounding the gland. **b** Many lymphocytes can be identified in further magnification with invasion into the altered gland (*arrow*)

multiple targeted and untargeted biopsies are still needed to verify and confirm the diagnosis. Sometimes, even additional molecular staining methods are necessary to establish the final diagnosis.

References

1. Banks PM (2007) Gastrointestinal lymphoproliferative disorders. Histopathology 50:42–54
2. Polglase AL, Fracs MS, Mc Laren W et al (2005) A fluorescence confocal endomicroscopy for in vivo microscopy of the upper and lower GI tract. Gastrointest Endosc 62:686–695
3. Leffler DA, Kelly CP (2006) Update on the evaluation and diagnosis of celiac disease. Curr Opin Allergy Clin Immunol (United States) 6:191–196
4. Dogan AM, Koulis A, Briskin MJ, Isaacson PG (1997) Expression of lymphocyte homing receptors and vascular addressins in low-grade gastric B-cell lymphomas of mucosa-associated lymphoid tissue. Am J Pathol 151:1361–1369
5. Cellier C, Patey N, Mauvieux L et al (1998) Abnormal intestinal intraepithelial lymphocytes in refractory sprue. Gastroenterology 114:471–481
6. Goldstein NS, Underhill J (2001) Morphologic features suggestive of gluten sensitivity in architecturally normal duodenal biopsy specimens. Am J Clin Pathol 116:63–71
7. Ranchod M, Lewin KJ, Dorfman RF (1978) Lymphoid hyperplasia of the gastrointestinal tract. A study of 26 cases and review of the literature. Am J Surg Pathol 2:383–400
8. O'Briain D, Kennedy M, Daly P et al (1989) Multiple lymphomatous polyposis of the gastrointestinal tract: a clinicopathologically distinctive form of non-Hodgkin's lymphoma of B-cell centrocytic type. Am J Surg Pathol 13:691–699
9. Banks PM, Chan J, Cleary ML et al (1992) Mantle cell lymphoma. A proposal for unification of morphologic, immunologic, and molecular data. Am J Surg Pathol 16:637–640
10. Wotherspoon AC, Doglioni C, Diss TC et al (1993) Regression of primary low-grade B-cell gastric lymphoma of mucosa-associated lymphoid tissue type after eradication of Helicobacter pylori. Lancet 342:575–577
11. Isaacson P, Wright DH (1983) Malignant lymphoma of mucosa-associated lymphoid tissue. A distinctive type of B-cell lymphoma. Cancer 52:1410–1416

7.5 Endomicroscopy of Colon Pathology

Ralf Kiesslich, Tomohiro Kato, Markus F. Neurath

Colorectal cancer is still one of the leading causes of cancer-related death in the Western world. Screening colonoscopy is widely accepted as the gold standard for early diagnosis of cancer. The prognosis for patients with colonic neoplasms is strictly dependent on the depth of infiltration and therefore depends on early detection of pre-invasive and neoplastic changes. Early detection makes it possible to cure the patient by means of immediate endoscopic resection.

In 2003, Sakashita et al. reported their initial experience with real-time confocal endoscopy in ex vivo specimens [1]. The prototype endomicroscope that was used (Olympus Optical Ltd., Tokyo, Japan) was passed through the working channel of an endoscope. The aim of the study was to establish new criteria for distinguishing between benign lesions and high-grade dysplasia or cancer. The study found a statistically significant difference between non-neoplastic and neoplastic lesions in relation to the detection rate of nuclei (dark areas) in laser-scanning confocal microscopy images.

On the basis of these results, the authors recommended preliminary criteria for a confocal imaging classification of high-grade intraepithelial neoplasia and cancer. Neoplasia was characterised by the presence of any structural abnormality and clear visualisation of nuclei. However, the sensitivity of this method for predicting neoplasms in the colorectum was only 60%, reflecting the limited resolution of the system that was used.

In a recently published study using the newly developed endomicroscopic system, 42 patients with indications for screening or surveillance colonoscopy after previous polypectomy underwent in vivo endomicroscopy with the confocal laser endoscope [2]. The aim of the study was to assess the histology in vivo during ongoing colonoscopy in order to diagnose intraepithelial neoplasias and colon cancer. Fluorescein-guided endomicroscopy of intraepithelial neoplasias and colon cancers showed a tubular, villous, or irregular architecture, with a reduced number of goblet cells. In addition, neovascularisation in neoplasms is characterised by irregular vessel architecture with fluorescein leakage.

A simple classification of the confocal pattern (◘ Table 7.2), based on initial experience with confocal endomicroscopy, was developed to allow differentiation between neoplastic and non-neoplastic tissue. Macroscopic and microscopic images were taken together to allow an immediate prediction of the histopathology. A total of 13 020 confocal images from 390 locations were compared with the histological data from 1038 biopsies [3]. It was possible to predict the presence of neoplastic changes using the newly developed confocal pattern classification with a sensitivity of 97.4%, a specificity of 99.4%, and an accuracy of 99.2% (◘ Figs. 7.16, 7.17).

Table 7.2. Endomicroscopic confocal pattern classification of colorectal lesions		
Grading	Vessel architecture	Crypt architecture
Normal	Hexagonal, honeycomb appearance that presents a network of capillaries outlining the stroma surrounding the luminal openings of the crypts	Regular luminal openings and distribution of crypts covered by a homogeneous layer of epithelial cells, including goblet cells
Regeneration	Hexagonal, honeycomb appearance with no increase or only a slight increase in the number of capillaries	Star-shaped luminal crypt openings or focal aggregation or regular-shaped crypts with a regular or reduced amount of goblet cells
Neoplasia	Dilated and distorted vessels with increased leakage; irregular architecture, with little or no orientation to the adjoining tissue.	Ridge-lined irregular epithelial layer with loss of crypts and goblet cells; irregular cell architecture, with little or no mucin

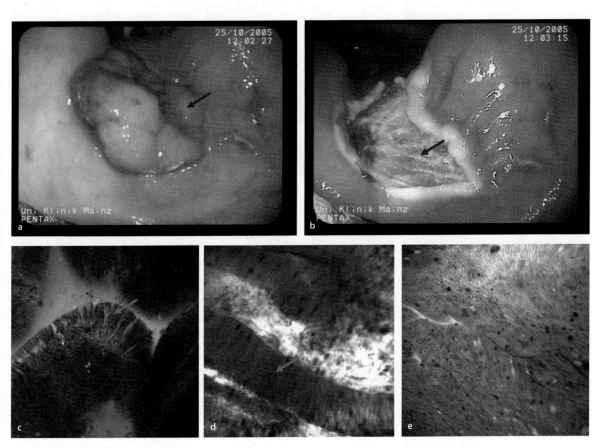

Fig. 7.16a–e. Endomicroscopy and resection of sporadic colorectal adenoma. **a** A broad-based lesion is visible right above the ileocaecal valve (*arrow*). **b** The lesion was resected en bloc after endomicroscopy. The muscularis propria becomes visible after endoscopic resection (*arrow*). **c** Endomicroscopy shows villous transformation of colonic architecture (*arrow*). **d** Adenomatous tissue is visible with depletion of goblet cells and columnar cell alignment (*arrow*). **e** Surface structure of adenomatous tissue. Some cells are irregular (*arrow*) and the intercellular spaces are wider than normal, leading to shine-through of fluorescence from the lamina propria

7

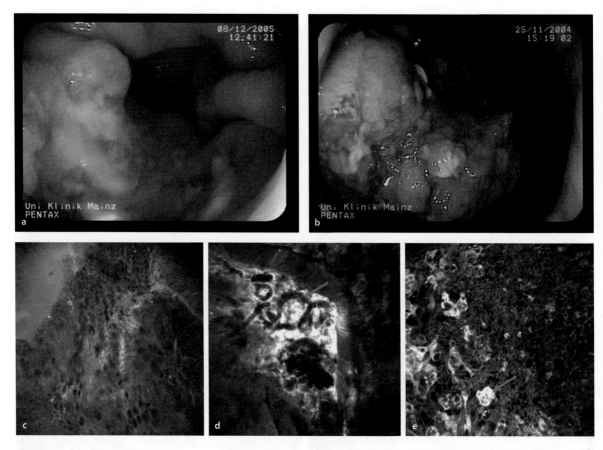

◘ Fig. 7.17a–e. Endomicroscopy of colorectal cancer. **a** A large cancerous lesion with ulceration is present in the sigmoid. **b** Another polypoid cancerous lesion shows spontaneous bleeding at the surface. **c** Endomicroscopy of a well differentiated adenocarcinoma with irregular cell architecture (*arrow*) can be seen. **d** Neoangiogenesis is characterised by the presence of irregular twisted vessels (*arrow*) with leakage of fluorescein into the surrounding tissue. **e** Cancer surface cells appear highly irregular, with gaps and vessels reaching the surface (*arrow*)

7.5.1 Ulcerative Colitis

It is not possible to examine the entire surface of the colon in the endomicroscopic mode. In patients with ulcerative colitis, it is therefore important to combine endomicroscopy with chromoendoscopy. Panchromoendoscopy with either methylene blue or indigo carmine is a valid diagnostic tool for improving the diagnostic yield of intraepithelial neoplasia using the »SURFACE« (◘ Table 7.3) recommendations [3]. Chromoendoscopy can reveal circumscribed lesions [4], and chromoscopy-guided confocal laser endomicroscopy can be used to predict intraepithelial neoplasias with a high degree of accuracy [5]. Targeted biopsies of relevant lesions can therefore be taken, and rapid confirmation of neoplastic changes using confocal laser endoscopy during colonoscopy may lead to significant improvements in the clinical management of patients with long standing ulcerative colitis (◘ Fig. 7.18).

In the first randomised trial of endomicroscopy, 153 patients with long-term ulcerative colitis who were in clinical remission were randomly assigned at a ratio of 1:1 to undergo either conventional colonoscopy or panchromoendoscopy using 0.1% methylene blue in conjunction

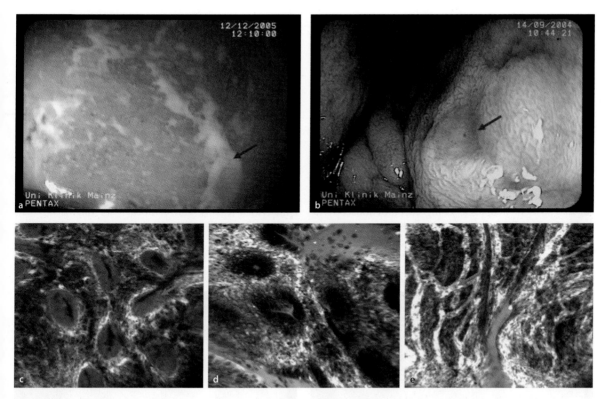

◪ Fig. 7.18a–e. Endomicroscopy of inflamed mucosa in ulcerative colitis. **a** Severe inflammatory changes are visible macroscopically. Longitudinal ulcerations (*arrow*) are present. **b** Chromoendoscopy with methylene blue highlights mucosal architecture, and small ulcerations become more prominent (*arrow*). **c** Endomicroscopy in patients with ulcerative colitis and mild inflammatory activity shows changes in crypt architecture. However, cell architecture within the crypts remains normal. Cellular inflammatory infiltrate leads to thickening of the lamina propria, and the intercryptal distance becomes larger. **d** Cryptal destruction is visible in more severe inflammatory changes (*arrow*). **e** Acute inflammation is characterised by the presence of increased vascularity (*arrow*) in combination with cryptal changes

◪ Table 7.3. SURFACE guidelines for chromoendoscopy in patients with ulcerative colitis

Strict patient selection	Patients with histologically proven ulcerative colitis who have been in clinical remission for at least 8 years. Avoid patients with active disease.
Unmasking of the mucosal surface	Excellent bowel preparation is needed. Remove mucus and remaining fluid in the colon when necessary.
Reduction of peristaltic waves	When the endoscope is drawn back, a spasmolytic agent should be used (if necessary).
Full-length staining of the colon	Perform full-length staining of the colon (panchromoendoscopy) in ulcerative colitis rather than local staining.
Augmented detection with dyes	Intravital staining with 0.4% indigo carmine or 0.1% methylene blue should be used to unmask flat lesions more frequently than with conventional colonoscopy.
Crypt architecture analysis	All lesions should be analysed according to the pit pattern classification. Whereas pit pattern types I–II suggest the presence of non-malignant lesions, staining patterns III–V suggest the presence of intraepithelial neoplasias and carcinomas.
Endoscopic targeted biopsies	Perform targeted biopsies of all mucosal alterations, particularly of circumscript lesions with staining patterns indicative of intraepithelial neoplasias and carcinomas (pit patterns III–V).

with endomicroscopy to detect intraepithelial neoplasia or colorectal cancer [5]. Circumscribed lesions in the colonic mucosa detected by chromoendoscopy were evaluated with endomicroscopy for cellular and vascular changes in accordance with the confocal pattern classification for predicting neoplasia. Targeted biopsies were taken from the areas examined and histologically graded according to the New Vienna classification.

In the standard colonoscopy group, randomised biopsies were taken every 10 cm between the anus and caecum, as well as targeted biopsies of visible mucosal changes. The primary outcome analysis was a histological diagnosis of neoplasia. Using chromoendoscopy in conjunction with endomicroscopy (80 patients, average examination time 42 min), significantly more intraepi-

thelial neoplasia was detected (19 versus four cases; $p=0.007$) than with standard colonoscopy (73 patients, average examination time 31 min). Endomicroscopy revealed different cellular structures (epithelial and blood cells), capillaries, and connective tissue limited to the mucosal layer. A total of 5580 confocal images from 134 circumscribed lesions were compared with the histological results from 311 biopsies. The presence of neoplastic changes was predicted with a high degree of accuracy (sensitivity 94.7 %, specificity 98.3 %, accuracy 97.8 %) [5] (◘ Fig. 7.19).

In summary, chromoendoscopy is able to reveal circumscribed lesions, and confocal laser microscopy can be used to confirm intraepithelial neoplasias with a high degree of accuracy. Biopsies can therefore be limited to

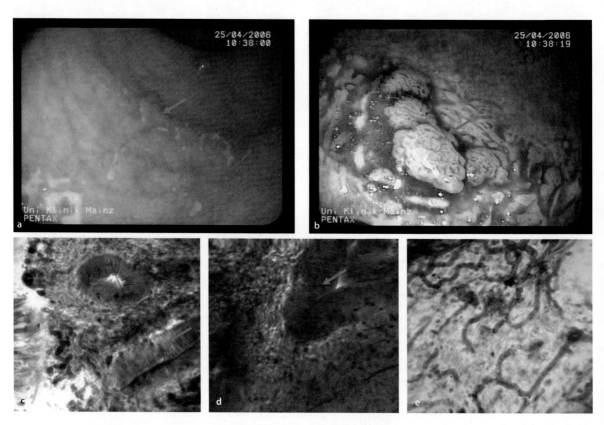

◘ **Fig. 7.19a–e.** Endomicroscopy of colitis-associated neoplasia. **a** The rectum is inflamed and an ulceration with partially elevated borders is present (*arrow*). **b** A suspected lesion can be identified after chromoendoscopy with methylene blue. A villous surface pattern becomes visible after staining. **c** Tubular architecture (*arrow*) can be seen in targeted endomicroscopy (*arrow*). **d** The cells are enlarged and a depletion of goblet cells is prominent. The overall shape and size of the crypts is irregular, which is highly suspicious for the presence of neoplastic changes. **e** The submucosa can be seen, which is rare, due to the limitation of imaging plane depth of the endomicroscopic system. However, here an increased vasculature is seen due to chronic inflammation within this area

targeted sampling of relevant lesions. In vivo histology with endomicroscopy may lead to significant improvements in the clinical management of patients with ulcerative colitis, with reduced numbers of biopsies being needed for confirmation of the condition and time being gained for immediate therapeutic intervention.

7.5.2 Microscopic Colitis

Microscopic colitis is a term used to define those clinicopathological entities characterised by chronic watery diarrhoea, normal radiological and endoscopic appearances, and microscopic abnormalities [6, 7]. Specific histopathological appearances can be used to further classify collagenous colitis, lymphocytic colitis and other conditions. Collagenous colitis differs from lymphocytic colitis by the presence of a subepithelial collagen band (≥10 μm) adjacent to the basal membrane. Both diseases present inflammatory changes in the lamina propria and superficial epithelial damage. Although microscopic colitis is considered a rare condition, increasing awareness of these entities among pathologists and clinicians has resulted in more frequent diagnosis. Their incidence is not well known; however, the incidence of lymphocytic colitis is about three times higher than that of collagenous colitis, and microscopic colitis should be considered as a major possibility in the work-up of chronic diarrhoea in older women [8].

Endomicroscopy makes it possible to locate and measure the distribution and thickness of collagenous bands underneath the epithelial layer, thus allowing targeted biopsies – a new approach in collagenous colitis, particularly in cases with disrupted subepithelial collagen deposits. At present, randomised biopsies are recommended, preferably from the right colon. The distribution of the collagenous bands can be patchy and segmental in the colon. Confocal endomicroscopy helps differentiate between affected and normal sites and can guide biopsies [9].

Also intraepithelial lymphocytes and an increased number of lymphocytes within the lamina propria of the right colon can be readily visualised, helping to verify the presence of lymphocytic colitis (◼ Fig. 7.20).

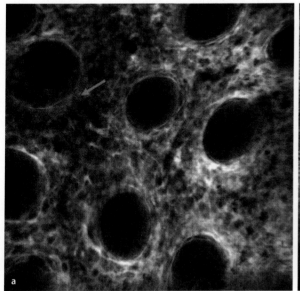
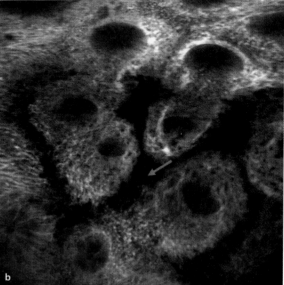

◼ **Fig. 7.20a,b.** Endomicroscopy of microscopic colitis. **a** Collagenous colitis is defined by the presence of collagenous bands in the lamina propria. Here, in addition, thickening of basement membrane is present. Targeted biopsy confirmed diagnosis of collagenous colitis. **a** Increased amount of lymphocytes leads to dark spots within the lamina propria. Single cells cannot be differentiated if multiple cells are present due to overlay of cells. However, this endomicroscopic feature (*arrow*) is quite specific for lymphocytic colitis, which was confirmed with endomicroscopic-guided biopsy

References

1. Sakashita M, Inoue H, Kashida J et al (2003) Virtual histology of colorectal lesions using laser-scanning confocal microscopy. Endoscopy 35:1033–1038
2. Kiesslich R, Burg J, Vieth M et al (2004) Confocal laser endoscopy for diagnosing intraepithelial neoplasias and colorectal cancer in vivo. Gastroenterology 127:706–713
3. Kiesslich R, Neurath MF (2004) Surveillance colonoscopy in ulcerative colitis: magnifying chromoendoscopy in the spotlight. Gut 53:165–167
4. Kiesslich R, Fritsch J, Holtmann M et al (2003) Methylene blue-aided chromoendoscopy for the detection of intraepithelial neoplasia and colon cancer in ulcerative colitis. Gastroenterology 124:880–888
5. Kiesslich R, Goetz M, Schneider C et al (2007) Confocal endomicroscopy as a novel method to diagnose colitis associated neoplasias in ulcerative colitis: a prospective randomized trial. Gastroenterology (in press)
6. Jawahari A, Talbot JC (1996) Microscopic and collagenous colitis. Histopathology 29:101–110
7. Bogomoletz WV (1994) Collagenous, microscopic and lymphocytic colitis. An evolving concept. Virchows Arch 424: 573–579
8. Fernández-Bañares F, Salas A, Forné M et al (1999) Incidence of collagenous and lymphocytic colitis: a 5-year population-based study. Am J Gastroenterol 94:418–423
9. Kiesslich R, Hoffman A, Goetz M et al (2006) In vivo diagnosis of collagenous colitis by confocal endomicroscopy. Gut 55:591–592

7.6 Endomicroscopy in Acute Graft-versus-Host Disease

Christian Bojarski, Jörg Carl Hoffmann, Martin Zeitz, Christoph Loddenkemper, Harald Stein

Infections and acute graft-versus-host disease (GvHD) are severe complications following allogeneic stem cell transplantation. GvHD commonly affects the skin, the gastrointestinal tract and the liver. The consequence of acute GvHD is the life-threatening destruction of vital organ functions.

Patients suspected to suffer from acute intestinal GvHD often present with diarrhoea, nausea and vomiting with abdominal pain or discomfort. In clinical practice it is of crucial importance to achieve a rapid diagnosis of GvHD in order to increase immunosuppressive therapy. Thus, biopsies of the gastrointestinal tract and/or the skin have to be performed to establish this diagnosis. Conventional histological examination using haematoxylin and eosin staining is the gold standard for diagnosing GvHD. According to the classification of Sale and Shulman [1, 2] acute GvHD can be assigned to a histological grade ranging from 1 to 4. The threshold for the minimum histopathological criteria of acute intestinal GvHD can be regarded as the presence of one apoptotic enterocyte per biopsy piece. Because apoptotic events are not restricted to the pathology of GvHD alone, immunohistochemical staining is added in selected cases to differentiate GvHD from other causes of apoptosis, such as CMV colitis.

Endoscopy of the rectum and sigmoid colon with subsequent biopsies is an easy method with minimal inconvenience for the patient. Patients with lesser degrees of intestinal GvHD often have only subtle macroscopic changes, while in the more severe variants of intestinal GvHD prominent colitis can usually be observed. When taking several biopsy samples of the colon one must be aware that after allogeneic stem cell transplantation patients have a higher risk of gastrointestinal bleeding due to thrombocytopoenia. For this reason they normally receive platelets before biopsies are taken.

Endomicroscopy of the lower gastrointestinal tract can help to obtain targeted biopsies of mucosal areas suspicious of GvHD (◘ Fig. 7.21). Therefore, it is necessary not only to inject fluorescein sodium 10% intravenously but also to apply acriflavine 0.05% topically with a spraying catheter through the working channel of the instrument. With acriflavine, it is possible to capture apoptosis of the crypt surface epithelial cells. It is difficult to clearly determine one single apoptotic cell and therefore to fulfil the minimal criteria for the diagnosis of GvHD during ongoing endomicroscopy. However, identification of several apoptotic cells in the surface epithelium and the beginning of the destruction of the crypt architecture, as well as maximum changes with a complete »crypt drop-out«, can be easily visualised during endomicroscopy. Moreover, endomicroscopy can help to reduce the amount of biopsy samples needed and therefore the risk of gastrointestinal bleeding in patients with haematological disorders.

In vivo confocal laser endomicroscopy is a newly developed diagnostic tool that allows virtual histology of the mucosal layer during ongoing endoscopy. The quality of the new, detailed images obtained with confocal laser endomicroscopy surely represents the start of a new era, in which this development in optical technology will allow unique visualisation of living cells and cellular structures at and below the surface of the gut. Several prospective studies have already been published confirming the high level of diagnostic accuracy of confocal laser endomicroscopy. The diagnostic spectrum of confocal

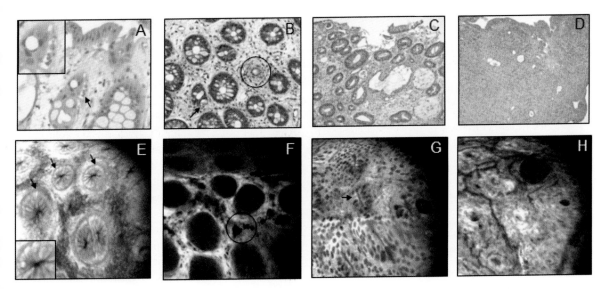

Fig. 7.21a–h. Endomicroscopy of graft-versus-host disease. **a–d** Histology (H&E., x 200), **e–h** (confocal endomicroscopy, 1024 x 1024 μm) in acute intestinal GvHD (sigmoid colon), classification of Sale and Shulman. GvHD I (**a, b, e, f**) with single apoptotic epithelial cells (*arrows*), intensified basal membrane (**e**) and focal epithelial regeneration (**b, f**, *circle*). GvHD II–III (**c, g**) with focal »crypt-drop-out« and single apoptoses (*arrow*), GvHD III–IV (**d, h**) with flattened mucosa. The normal crypt architecture is completely abolished

endomicroscopy is currently expanding from screening and surveillance for colorectal cancer to include Barrett's oesophagus, *Helicobacter pylori*-associated gastritis, and gastric cancers. In addition, several other indications – such as coeliac disease, microscopic colitis, mucosa-associated lymphoid tissue (MALT) lesions, GvHD and squamous-cell carcinoma – are also being investigated. Endomicroscopy is likely to play an increasingly important diagnostic role during gastrointestinal endoscopy in the future and can currently be used to avoid random biopsies and focus on targeted biopsies. Further technological developments and improvements are likely to enhance the imaging facilities further.

References

1. Sale et al (1979) Gastrointestinal graft-versus-host disease in man. A clinicopathologic study of the rectal biopsy. Am J Surg Pathol. 3 (4): 291–299
2. Shulman et al (2006) Histopathologic diagnosis of chronic graft-versus-host disease: National Institutes of Health Consensus Development Project on Criteria for Clinical Trials in Chronic Graft-versus-Host Disease: II. Pathologic Working Group Report. Biol Blood Marrow Transplant. 12 (1): 31–47

Live Tissue Imaging with Conventional Confocal Microscopy

Marshall H. Montrose, Alastair J.M. Watson

Key concepts:

- Bench-top confocal microscopy is an essential partner in both optimizing and defining what the confocal endoscope should report.
- A new window for translational research has opened that allows firm comparison of outcomes from living tissues of man and mammalian model systems using the same imaging technology.

The advanced technologies incorporated into confocal endoscopes are based on an established foundation of experience in confocal microscopy. This chapter will review some of the basics of confocal microscopy and highlight the complementary capabilities that such microscopes can provide compared with confocal endoscopy.

8.1 A Primer on Laser-Scanning Confocal Imaging

The underlying technology of confocal imaging was pioneered by Marvin Minsky in 1957, as a means to visualise cells in three dimensions. With the advent of cheap powerful computers and lasers in the early 1980s, the first commercial instruments were introduced, and confocal microscopy rapidly became a routine tool for biological research.

The physics of fluorescence drive the design of all fluorescence microscopes, including confocal instruments. Fluorescence is the light emitted by a molecule (a fluor-phore) in response to absorbing light of a different colour. A fundamental property is that the emitted light is always of a lower energy (longer wavelength) than the excitation light that is absorbed. For example, when the excitation light is blue (450–500 nm wavelength),the emitted light may be green (500–550 nm) or red (600–700 nm). The preferred colours of both excitation and emission are a matter of personality of the individual fluorophores, and there is a desirable diversity of fluorescent indicators that can be used singly or in combination because of their different colours.

Confocal imaging is a clever way of viewing fluorescence from a thin region within a thick specimen, without the need to physically slice up the specimen. This is called optical sectioning. In laser-scanning confocal instruments, the spot of exciting light from a laser is steered systematically across the sample by moving mirrors. This helps localise excitation to a restricted spot at any given time, but because the emitted light travels deeply thru the specimen while the laser points at any given spot, this alone is not able to provide optical sectioning. If only laser scanning is used, the reported fluorescence produces sharp images only if the specimen is very thin; in the range of 1–5 μm. Blurred images result from thicker samples.

The key to understanding the next step in how a confocal microscope works is to understand why thick samples produce blurred images in conventional fluorescence microscopes. Let us take as an example light rays passing though a series of lenses to produce an image in the eye. A ray of light that arises from the plane of focus of the lens system will produce a sharp image at the eyepiece. A ray of light that arises from above the plane of focus of the lens system also enters the eyepiece but is out of focus because it arose from outside the plane of focus. Such a situation will occur if a fluorescent sample is examined which is thicker than the plane of focus of the optics of the microscope. Both the in-focus light (at the focal plane of the microscope) and the out-of-focus light (above and below the focal plane) will contribute to the image, causing the image to be blurred and indistinct.

In a confocal microscope the in-focus light is selectively allowed to reach the fluorescence detectors, in preference to the out-of-focus light. The key component is a pinhole placed in the emission light path right before the fluorescence detectors, at a locale where the emission light is focused at a **con**jugate **focal** plane. At this locale for the confocal pinhole, the in-focus emission light passes through the pinhole efficiently, but out-of-focus emission light is *not* focused at the pinhole, and so a much lower fraction of the out-of-focus light is able to pass through and reach the detector. While this simple expedient of adding a pinhole to the light path helps to solve the problem of blurred images from thick samples, the confocal pinhole strategy has its limitations. If the fluorescence from the focal plane is much lower than the fluorescence from the out-of-focus regions, the pinhole may not be able to discard enough out-of-focus light to make the desired fluorescence the brightest item in the image (◘ Fig. 8.1). A new strategy, called two-photon microscopy, can push beyond this limit. It is discussed in Sect. 8.4.

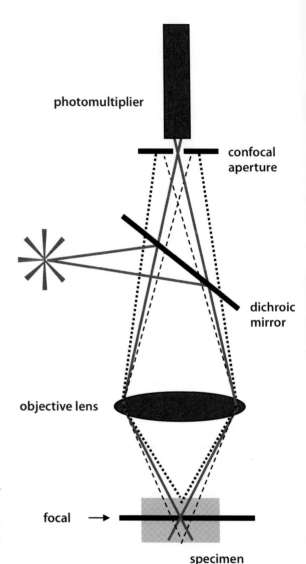

◘ **Fig. 8.1.** Diagram of a confocal microscope (Reprinted from Gastroenterology, 129(3), A.J.M. Watson, S. Chu, L. Sieck, O. Gerasimenko, T. Bullen, F. Campbell, M. McKenna, T. Rose, and M.H. Montrose. Epithelial barrier function in vivo is sustained despite gaps in epithelial layers, 902-12, 2005, with permission from Elsevier)

8.2   Imaging Fixed Versus Living Tissue

While confocal microscopy is now the standard tool for analysis of dead, fixed fluorescent specimens, it has been less commonly applied to living specimens. In early confocal microscopy designs, this was largely because the amount of excitation light power needed to resolve

confocal fluorescence was enough to damage cells within just a few images. As the light economy of microscopes improved (better detectors, better light path, etc.), live cell and live tissue imaging became possible. While there are uncontested strengths and reasons for fixed tissue imaging, the emergence of live tissue confocal imaging has resulted in insights that were not possible previously.

The major advantages of live tissue imaging stem from the abilities to examine intact complex structures and to image changing events over time. As discussed previously, optical sectioning allows high-resolution imaging of regions that were previously accessible only by physically carving up a specimen. As one focuses into regions within a tissue, retaining cell-cell contacts and the diversity of cell types in their natural habitat can result in some surprising features of cellular function that would be missed in other experimental formats. From our own experience, we have reported that the complex cellular architecture of native tissue produces areas of limited mixing in both stomach and colon. The result is the creation of microdomains of function in the extracellular spaces that can be directly visualised, and their contribution to tissue function can be evaluated. The additional strength of being able to evaluate the dynamics of cell and tissue function over time provides insights into cellular responsiveness without needing to dissociate or isolate specific cell types.

Live tissue imaging does not come without a price and requires extra considerations. Firstly, any fluorophore (dye) you intend to use must be able to penetrate to the site of interest. This is readily tested by finding the right spot and seeing if your dye is able to reach it reliably, and by working with a selection of dyes to find the best one. Secondly, when multiple images are created over time in an environment with oxygen, high light exposure can cause both destruction of your reporter dye (photobleaching) and damage to your cells, as photobleaching can release free radicals and other toxic by-products. This is mitigated by always starting live cell imaging with maximal detector sensitivity (usually indicated as detector »gain«) and the lowest possible laser power. If the image is not good enough for your purposes, then you have to figure out the best scientific compromise. You can get a brighter image by getting more light to the detector by opening the pinhole (thicker optical section), or by raising laser power while checking to make sure no damage occurs. You can get a less noisy image by averaging multiple scans for each time point or using some of the other suggested strategies to allow you to lower detector gain. Using these guidelines, it is possible to put small whole organs or even anaesthetised small animals on the stage of a confocal microscope and obtain microscopic images of living, functioning tissue with subcellular resolution.

There are hundreds of fluorophores that can be used for biological research, and most of them can be used for live tissue work, either in their current format or after some adjustment. Some synthetic fluorescent molecules, such as fluorescein-5-isothiocyanate (FITC), can be conjugated to antibodies or other molecules and used as a fluorophore that reports location of a binding protein target. In vivo studies with whole organs or whole animals are possible, providing that the antibody recognises a surface epitope on a protein or is directed against a circulating factor. Other synthetic fluorophores can readily enter cells in vivo and bind to specific cellular components. A number of dyes such as Hoechst 33342, acridine orange and ethidium bromide bind to nucleic acids and are commonly used to image cellular nuclei in confocal microscopy. Aside from nuclei, other intracellular organelles can be specifically labelled with fluorescent dyes, such as mitochondria with rhodamine 123 and the Golgi apparatus with dyes conjugated to ceramide derivatives. Perhaps most exciting is the ability to create transgenic animals in which the expression of fluorescent proteins [of the enhanced green fluorescent protein (EGFP) family or others] can be driven by cell-type-specific promoters to report the location of specific cell types, or the fluorescent protein can be fused to an intrinsic cellular protein to report on the locale of the fusion protein.

Other applications of confocal imaging include detecting cell movement or cell migration within solid tissues. Blood vessels can be easily imaged with dyes such as fluorescein, and leucocytes can be imaged with antibodies conjugated to probes such as Texas Red, which emit light at a different wavelength. With the use of narrow-pass optical filters the two dyes can be imaged separately or together in the same image.

Laser light delivers high energy to fluorescence probes which, if prolonged, will cause bleaching. Some experimental protocols take advantage of this property to measure diffusion rates within the cytoplasm of cells. If a small area of cytoplasm is bleached with a spot of very bright laser light, the rate at which the fluorescence recovers can be measured. The fluorescence will be restored by diffusion of unbleached dye into the bleached area and will give a measure of diffusion within the cell or tissue.

Some fluorescence probes that are highly cell impermeable can be used as permeability probes of epithelial tissue. For example, the permeability of tissue to dextran conjugated to FITC can be used to determine sites of permeation in intestinal tissue.

It is sometimes not necessary to label cells at all, as they contain intrinsically fluorescent substances such as NADH, which can be imaged at the appropriate wavelengths on the confocal microscope. NADH fluorescence has been used to report on cell viability and metabolic status in both pancreas and muscle. Sometimes fluorescence is not even required. By examining the confocal reflectance of laser excitation light (the light that simply bounces off a tissue) it is possible to gain structural information from any recognisable cell or structure that has a reflective surface (e.g. cellular organelles) with subcellular resolution.

Finally, there is an ever-expanding range of synthetic dyes and fluorescent proteins whose fluorescence proper-

ties change in proportion to some cellular function. The classic examples of such reporter dyes are Fura-2 and fluo-3 which bind to calcium ions, or BCECF which binds hydrogen ions. In a clever application of cellular chemistry (first used by Ephraim Racker in the late 1970s), such dyes are often built to include an attached acetoxymethyl ester group (◘ Fig. 8.2). This group shields the charge of a carboxy (COO-) group and makes the molecules membrane permeable so that they enter cells. Once inside the cell, the acetoxymethyl group is cleaved off by cytoplasmic esterases (expressed in virtually all cells) to often render the molecule both more brightly fluorescent and membrane impermeable so that it remains trapped inside the cell.

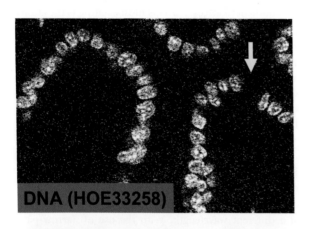

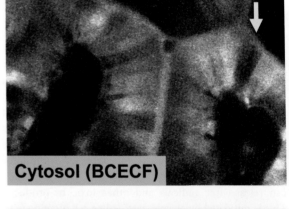

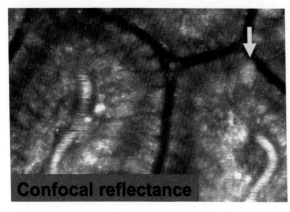

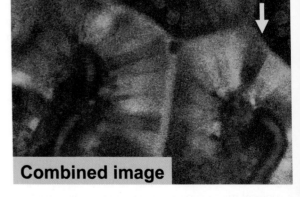

◘ **Fig. 8.2.** Small intestinal epithelium. The nuclei of villus epithelial cells are stained with Hoechst 33258. A gap in the epithelium is indicated by an *arrow* (*top left*). Cytosol of villus epithelium stained with BCECF administered in the acetoxymethyl ester form (*top right*). Confocal reflectance showing reflective material in the gap in the epithelial monolayer (*bottom right*). All three images are combined with nuclei in blue, cytosol in green and confocal reflectance in red. (Taken from [1])

8.3   Going from Qualitative to Quantitative

The most desirable reporter dyes change colour (of either excitation or emission) proportional to the magnitude of the cellular function they sense. Fura-2, for example, can be excited at two wavelengths, 340 and 380 nm with a single emission wavelength of 510 nm. As the concentration of calcium rises, the intensity of emission at 340 nm excitation rises while the intensity at 380 nm falls. The advantage of such a situation is that the ratio of fluorescence seen in response to these two excitation wavelengths (340 nm fluorescence/380 nm fluorescence) can be used to measure calcium concentration. When the Fura-2 ratio is measured for each spot (pixel) in an image separately, the resulting ratio image can report heterogeneity in cellular calcium. If the quantification of the ratio is done correctly, the major advantage is that the ratio value is a faithful reporter of the cellular function independent of dye concentration, changes in concentration when dye leaks from the cell, and cell or tissue motion.

The requirements for such quantitative imaging are not many, but they are stringent. All pixels in an image must be on scale, with an image defined as a matrix of numbers (pixels) that report intensity. So if you have something that is too bright and it simply saturates the brightness under your image settings, any such bright pixels are useless for quantification. Just as important, any background fluorescence (e.g. the image you collect when you focus out of your specimen) must also be something greater than zero intensity (black in the image). The second requirement is that if you are going to do ratio imaging, you have to collect both the numerator and the denominator image quickly so that you can be reasonably sure that tissue has not moved and that the cellular value you want to follow has not changed much in the time it took you to collect the two images. The final requirement is that if you are imaging a living moist tissue, you must use an objective lens that uses water as the solution between the lens and sample. This ensures that fluorescence will not diminish unpredictably as you focus deeper into the tissue. Starting from these three principle requirements, it will be possible to get reliable data for quantification.

8.4   Moving Beyond Confocal Imaging

Although confocal microscopy represents a large advance over conventional microscopy, some disadvantages remain. The excitation light delivered to the specimen will penetrate and excite fluorophores throughout the illuminated specimen. This means that high light energy is delivered to large depths of the tissue, which can cause dispersed photobleaching and in some cases tissue damage. Another limitation is that the maximum depth at which a focal plane can be obtained is limited to 250 μm in organs such as the liver. This is because of scattering of photons by cells as they travel to and from the focal plane. In some tissues where cell nuclei are very dense, such as the intestinal epithelium, depth of focal plane is further restricted to approximately 60 μm.

These shortcomings are circumvented by a newer technology called 2-photon microscopy, which can create optical sections at depths of up to 1 mm and causes much less photobleaching in a thick specimen. The theoretical basis of 2-photon microscopy was established by Maria Goeppert-Mayer in her doctoral thesis in 1931. She showed that two low-energy photons, as opposed to a single high-energy photon, can excite a fluorescence molecule, causing emission of light. This concept was incorporated into microscopy by Watt Webb's group at Cornell University in 1990 by using a laser pulsing at 80 Mhz with a pulse length of 100 femtoseconds. This gives the very high flux of photons required for simultaneous absorption of two photons by the fluorphore. The only point in the light path where there is a high probability of simultaneous absorption of two photons is at the focal plane of the microscope. Thus an optical section is created without the use of a pinhole, and the light absorption that results in photobleaching is restricted to the focal plane. Light energy emitted from the fluorphore comes only from the focal plane (the only site of light absorption that results in fluorescence) and so confocal pinholes are not needed. An important benefit is that this also allows deep tissue imaging because there is no battle to resolve the in-focus fluorescence from a deep contaminating ocean of out-of-focus fluorescence. Further improvements in deep tissue focusing come from the use of infra-red lasers with low energy photons. This results in less light scattering within the tissue than with the high-energy (short-wavelength) excitation used in conventional confocal microscopes. To date, 2-photon microscopy has not been incorporated into an endoscope, but the advantages make this a likely event in the future.

8.5 Selecting the Correct Instrument for the Task at Hand

Both confocal endoscopy and confocal microscopy have the capability to report events from native tissues. Apart from the obvious need to use endoscopy when approaching tissues still within human patients, there are a number of features of the two types of devices that encourage selection of one or the other. There are three devices that will be considered. One is the conventional confocal microscope that has been the main focus of this chapter. Second is the confocal endoscope that is gaining popularity. Third is a recently introduced device that utilises the same miniaturised scanner as in the Pentax confocal endoscope but is designed as a hand-held confocal probe (a pen confocal; Optiscan model Five-1).

8.5.1 Translational Research Ability

There are some research questions in which it would be an advantage to use the same scanner in human and animal studies to assure reliable translation of work in one system to the other. While it is possible to try to homogenise imaging parameters between a conventional confocal microscope and the confocal endoscope, life is made easier if the same scanner can be used in both experimental modes. This is now possible with the Optiscan Five 1 system in combination with the Pentax confocal endoscope.

8.5.2 Multicolour Fluorescence

As discussed above, there is often a need to perform ratiometric measures, or to co-localise different fluorophores as a means to explore the location of distinct proteins in the same cell. This is currently possible only with conventional confocal microscopy. In such microscopes the use of appropriate optical filters and multiple detectors make it simple to visualise the two colours of emitted light simultaneously or in rapid sequence.

8.5.3 Maximal Subcellular Resolution

The confocal endoscope and pen confocal have amazing resolution, but the optical section of ~7-μm thickness and 0.7-μm lateral resolution is fixed. In conventional confocal microscopy this resolution can be improved two- to threefold through the use of alternative objectives.

8.5.4 Wide Field of View and Sporadic Events/Structures

In studies of isolated native tissues, especially of diseased tissue, there is often unpredictable heterogeneity within the sample. This is difficult to systematically scan with a conventional confocal microscope because it has only a limited field of view. The pen confocal is a simple hand-held system to rapidly scan over large areas of tissue at good resolution and has an extremely large field of view for the magnification, which is better than conventional objective lenses in current commercially available confocal microscopes.

8.5.5 More Flexible Imaging Parameters in Confocal Microscopy

While the Five-1 scanner provides outstanding light sensitivity and good spatial resolution, it can report only a single channel of fluorescence and it is designed for simple collection of images across the focal plane (i.e. XY image plane). If your needs are for higher (or lower) spatial resolution or scanning speed, you will need to go to conventional confocal microscopy. Similarly, conventional confocal microscopy gives great flexibility in imaging parameters such as direct imaging through the focal plane (XZ plane imaging), more reliable and quantifiable z-axis motion control, and automated image collection in both time and space (◘ Fig. 8.3).

8.6 Conclusion

Bench-top confocal microscopy has strengths that complement what can be learned by confocal endoscopy and should be viewed as an essential partner in both optimising and defining what the confocal endoscope reports. In this way, a new window for translational research has opened that allows firm comparisons of outcomes from living tissues of man and mammalian model systems using the same technology.

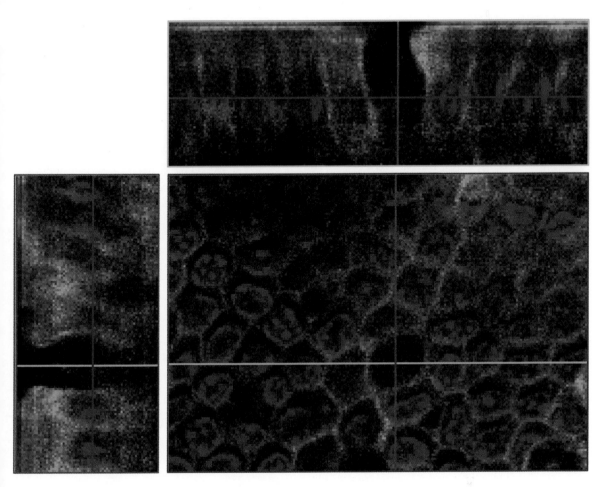

◘ Fig. 8.3. Three-dimensional reconstruction of mouse small intestinal epithelium. The cytosol is stained with transgenically expressed yellow fluorescent protein shown in green. The nuclei are stained with Hoechst 33258 in blue. The two views from the side are computer constructions from 50 images taken in the en face view 0.5 μm apart

Reference

1. Watson AJ, Chu S, Sieck L, Gerasimenko O, Bullen T, Campbell F, McKenna M, Rose T, Montrose MH (2005) Epithelial barrier function *in vivo* is sustained despite gaps in epithelial layers. Gastroenterology 129 (3):902–912. Fig. 1, DEFG panels. Fig. 2A

Functional and Molecular Imaging with Confocal Laser Endomicroscopy

Martin Goetz, Ralf Kiesslich, Markus F. Neurath, Alastair J.M. Watson

Key concepts:
- Changes of vessels architecture and neovascularisation in tumor tissues can be easily analyzed by endomicroscopy.
- Endomicroscopy can also be used to analyze surface receptors in the GI tract and may be used in the future for functional and molecular imaging in man.

9.1 Aims of Functional and Molecular Imaging

In vivo functional and molecular imaging is an emerging new field in gastroenterology. Ex vivo histopathological examination of tissue specimens offers a snapshot view into the tissue, capturing the moment at which the biopsy has been taken. The specimen is subjected to the fixation and staining process, making it prone to artefact. In vivo imaging with confocal endomicroscopy, however, offers the possibility of dynamic monitoring of the living tissue without the need for fixation. To our current knowledge, staining with intravenous fluorescein sodium or topical acriflavine hydrochloride does not alter tissue properties in a way that could influence biological processes. Therefore, with confocal endomicroscopy, a time axis inherent to biological processes can be added to a mere morphological visualisation at a given time point. In this way, confocal endomicroscopy is quite analogous to continuous macroscopic imaging by ultrasonography, providing dynamic microscopic imaging of perfusion and cellular and subcellular function.

Immunohistochemistry makes diagnostic use of the molecular properties of cells. In a multistep procedure, the specimen is incubated with antibodies directed against the molecule of interest. Secondary antibodies against the primary antibody are added and, in a further step, linked to a colour-generating chemical that indicates the presence of the molecule of interest upon light or fluorescence microscopic examination. This ex vivo staining procedure is often used for the molecular classification of suspected malignant disease. It requires the endoscopist to biopsy a lesion that is detected by other means than by its molecular properties.

It would greatly enhance the value of endoscopy if the endoscopist were able to reliably predict the malignant potential of a lesion based on its morphological, functional and molecular characteristics. This would permit immediate diagnosis and therapy, such as endoscopic resection, and potentially could enable prediction and evaluation of response to targeted molecular therapy.

9.2 Functional Imaging

Functional imaging with confocal endomicroscopy uses both morphological and functional criteria for tissue evaluation to visualise dynamic processes, as outlined above.

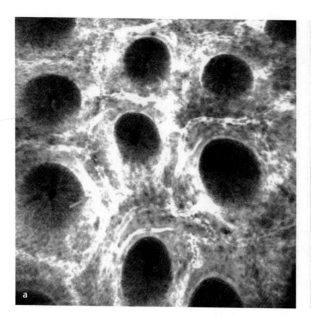
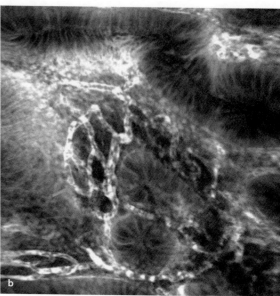

□ **Fig. 9.1a,b.** Changes of vessel architecture and function in ulcerative colitis. Active inflammation is suspected in areas that show enhanced vessel leakiness or increased vasculature. In a extravasation of fluorescein (*arrows*) indicates disturbed capillary function, while in b the number and tortuosity of the vessels are predominantly increased

It is used for imaging of perfusion and perfusion changes, cell shedding, cell migration, necrosis and apoptosis.

Capillary function is altered in inflammation and in neoplasia. With confocal endomicroscopy, this can be assessed in several ways, combining the appreciation of an increase in the number of vessels in the mucosa and their shape with the evaluation of capillary function. In inflammation, the vessels are increased both in number and leakiness, but the vessel diameter is usually of regular size. The enhanced extravasation of fluorescein is characteristic of active mucosal inflammation, such as in ulcerative colitis. A bright contrast is seen in the lamina propria that is not confined to vessel structures. Often, an inflammatory infiltration of the lamina propria is seen along with the enhanced leakiness (□ Fig. 9.1a). In a post-inflammatory state, a mere increase in the number of capillaries without significant dye leakage can be seen (□ Fig. 9.1b).

In neoplasia, neoangiogenesis has been appreciated as a paramount step in the pathogenesis of tumours. Tumour vessels differ from capillaries in healthy tissue, as they show an enhanced leakiness and a tortuous, irregular structure and diameter, both of which are not readily visible on conventional ex vivo staining. Since fluorescein does not stain nuclei, typical histological features of neoplasia such as an altered nuclear-to-cytoplasmic ratio and chromatin condensation cannot be evaluated in vivo after fluorescein injection. Therefore, visualisation of vessel structure and function gives important clues for the in vivo diagnosis. In high-grade intraepithelial neoplasia and carcinoma, the vessels are irregularly dilated and show enhanced permeability for fluorescein that visibly leaks into the tissue (□ Fig. 9.2a).

In animal models of human diseases, continuous monitoring of perfusion is achieved more easily, as staining protocols using other fluorescent dyes yield additional information about vessel structure and function. *Lycopersicon esculentum* lectin is a lectin that binds to glycoprotein moieties on endothelial cells. Staining of tumour vessels with FITC-labelled *L. esculentum* lectin visualised the inhomogeneity of the glycoprotein expression on tumour vessel endothelium by a weak and patchy staining of capillary walls upon in vivo confocal microscopy (□ Fig. 9.2b). Passive permeation of dye into malignant tissue identified leaky tumour vessels in liver metastases in extended disease [1]. Assessment of vessel leakiness has also been used to identify necrotic tissue by extravasation of FITC-labelled high-molecular-weight dextrans that are usually retained within the circulation in intact tissue.

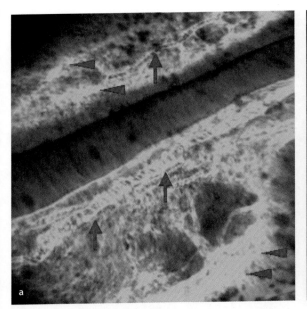 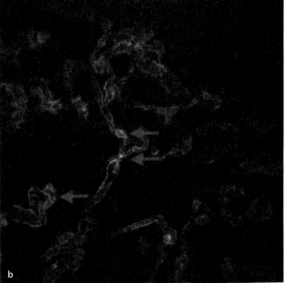

Fig. 9.2a,b. Neoangiogenesis. **a** Although the epithelial layer is still contained by the basal membrane in this optical section, the vessel structure and function are indicative of high-grade malignancy. Vessels are of irregular diameter (*arrows*), and leakage of fluorescein into the tissue is significantly increased (*arrowheads*). Histopathology confirmed the presence of an invasive rectal carcinoma. **b** In a murine tumour model (HEK-293 cells), tumour vessels show an irregular distribution of endothelial glycoproteins as mirrored in a patchy staining pattern (*arrows*) after intravenous injection of FITC-labelled *L. esculentum* lectin that is bound by N-acetylglucosamine oligomers on endothelial cells. Tumour vessels are tortuous and have a corkscrew appearance. (Edge length: 500 μm)

However, these staining protocols are not yet registered for clinical use in patients.

Ex vivo labelling of single cells has been exploited diagnostically in scintigraphic imaging of inflammation (leucocytes) and bleeding sources (erythrocytes). In animal models, ex vivo FITC-labelling of erythrocytes and reinjection has permitted visualisation of the blood flow by confocal in vivo microscopy and – combined with blood plasma staining – was able to identify perfusion anomalies such as a microthrombosis in vivo by observation of a stop in plasma and blood cell flow within the vessel [2]. Similarly, labelling of white blood cells that can be visualised by in vivo confocal microscopy is possible in animal models and has permitted observation of leucocyte–endothelium interactions such as homing to the vessel wall in animals. Although these methods are currently to be considered experimental, it is conceivable that these labelling techniques that are already used in radiographic procedures could also be used for microscopic tissue diagnosis by confocal endomicroscopy. This will permit observation of cell interactions in their natural environment in human beings in vivo and could potentially greatly enhance our understanding of biological processes in many diseases.

Apart from the visualisation of vessel function, confocal endomicroscopy has also been used to describe subtle features of the function of normal human intestinal epithelium that seem to be very sensitive to fixation procedures. Recently, distinct gaps in the intact epithelial layer have been described [3]. These gaps seem to arise after the shedding of apoptotic cells. In apoptotic cells, the nucleus is condensed and therefore brighter than nuclei in adjacent cells after topical staining with acriflavine [4]. The basal orientation is lost before the cell is repelled from the epithelial layer (□ Fig. 9.3). These features of apoptosis and epithelial regeneration can hardly be seen in conventional ex vivo histopathology and are difficult to distinguish from shrinking artefacts. In animal models, where longer observation times are possible, apoptosis of single cells and shedding become visible, illustrating the necessity of in vivo imaging of cells in their natural surroundings to adequately describe biological processes.

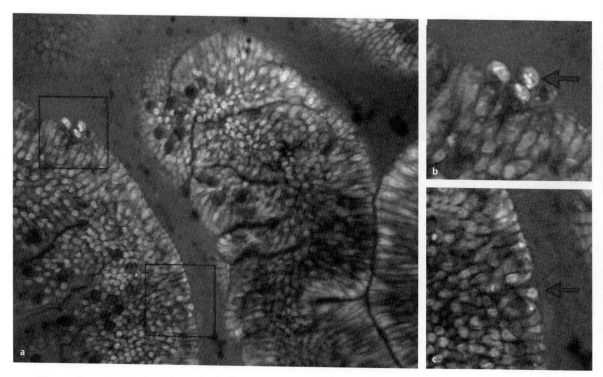

▫ Fig. 9.3a–c. Gaps in the gut and apoptosis. Following topical acriflavine administration, the surface epithelial layer of the duodenal villi is stained (**a**). Within the regular orientation of epithelial cells, three cell nuclei are condensed and fragmented in cells which are about to be shed (**b**), indicating apoptosis. In **c**, a single cell within the cellular lining shows a loss of the basal nuclear orientation and retraction from the adjacent epithelial cells. These changes are part of the normal regenerative processes of the intestinal epithelium. (Edge length: **a** 500 μm)

9.3   Molecular Imaging

The goal of molecular imaging is to identify and characterise cells by the molecules they express. Targeting of molecules that allow early detection and rapid identification of malignancies and their precursor lesions is highly desirable. Potential molecular targets of such an approach are growth factor receptors or tyrosine kinases that are frequently over-expressed in malignant tissue. Their major role for tumour growth has been exemplified by the therapeutic efficacy of imatinib mesylate and epidermal growth factor receptor (EGFR)- or vascular endothelial growth factor (VEGF)-targeted antibody therapy.

In animals, in vivo molecular imaging by confocal microscopy has already been achieved. Following injection of a fluorescently labelled octreotate that binds to somatostatin receptors, somatostatin receptor positive cells have been selectively highlighted. This permitted the identification of neuroendocrine tumour cells and pancreatic endocrine cells and exemplifies the in vivo visualisation of cell types in their natural surrounding, based on their molecular properties. Following injection of the labelled molecule, even such detailed analysis as observation of cell surface binding, internalisation of the dye and renal excretion was possible by confocal microscopy in a living organism, illustrating the visualisation of molecular events in vivo [1]. Anikajenko et al used an FITC antibody to human avb3 integrin complex (vitronectin receptor,expressed in high levels on melanoma cells) to enable in vivo microscopy of human melonoma cells xenografed into nude mice. These studies demonstrate that in vivo molecular imaging by confocal endomicroscopy can be achieved and is able to identify malignant cells (▫ Fig. 9.4a).

In human beings, only ex vivo examinations have been performed so far for molecular imaging. It has been shown that fluorescent staining of resected human colon

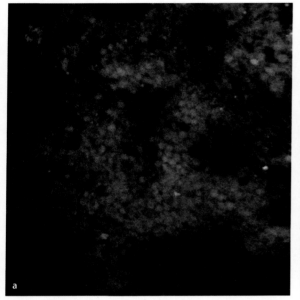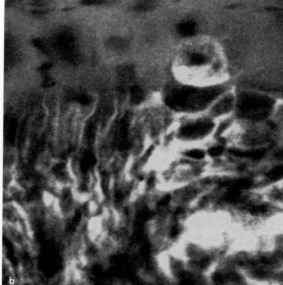

Fig. 9.4a,b. a In vivo molecular imaging following administration of a fluorescently labelled ligand to somatostatin receptor of a neuroendocrine tumour in the mouse shows a patchy distribution of receptor-positive tumour cells within the tumour tissue. The targeted staining highlights malignant cells in vivo that are detected by confocal microscopy and were subsequently confirmed by conventional immunohistochemistry. Images were captured with a hand-held confocal laparoscopy probe (FIVE1, Optiscan, Australia) that employs scanning devices identical to those of the confocal endomicroscope (Pentax EC-3870CIFK). **b** Ex vivo molecular staining of a resected human colon adenoma contrasts malignant cells after topical application of a FITC-labelled antibody to EGFR. Images were captured with the Pentax confocal endomicroscope. This illustrates that molecular imaging can be achieved in human beings even after topical dye administration. (Edge length: **a** 400 µm, **b** 250 µm)

adenoma specimens yields sufficient contrast for confocal endomicroscopy after topical staining with a fluorescently labelled antibody against EGFR (**❑** Fig. 9.4b). Similarly, incubation of biopsies with an anti-CD44v6-antibody identified aberrant crypt foci based on their surface molecule expression [5]. Therefore, it might be assumed that topical staining for molecular alterations such as receptor over-expression could also be possible in human beings in vivo. This could be exploited for diagnosis of neoplasia and inflammation, but also to predict response to targeted molecular therapy in inflammation and cancer by the intensity of target expression.

For application in human beings, the route of dye delivery (i.e. topical or intravenous) has not yet been evaluated. Topical administration onto the mucosa would probably be favourable to patient safety and ease of user applicability. However, the development of specific molecular tracers still needs thorough evaluation as to specificity, sensitivity and safety in animal models, before in vivo application in human subjects is conceivable. Yet the current data suggest that fluorescent labelling of molecules that are ideally present only on target (e.g. malignant) cells can be achieved in vivo in human beings. This complements morphological imaging to offer cellular identification with high specificity and sensitivity – in combination with macroscopic fluorescent imaging, a red-flag technique for identifying and characterising areas of interest and potentially predicting response to therapy.

References

1. Goetz M, Fottner C, Schirrmacher E, Delaney P, Gregor S, Schneider C, Strand D, Kanzler S, Memadathil B, Weyand E, Holtmann M, Schirrmacher R, Weber MM, Anlauf M, Klöppel G, Vieth M, Galle PR, Bartenstein P, Neurath MF, Kiesslich R. In vivo confocal real

time mini-microscopy in animal models of human inflammatory and neoplastic diseases. Endoscopy 2007; 39(4):350–6

2.   Goetz M, Thomas S, Delaney P, Schneider C, Kempski O, Gregor S, Galle, PR, Neurath, MF, Kiesslich, R (2006) Dynamic imaging of vessels and perfusion by hand-held confocal laser microscopy. J Vasc Res 43:40–40 [Suppl 1]

3.   Watson AJ, Chu S, Sieck L, Gerasimenko O, Bullen T, Campbell F, McKenna M, Rose T, Montrose MH (2005) Epithelial barrier function in vivo is sustained despite gaps in epithelial layers. Gastroenterology 129:902–912

4.   Watson AJ, Kiesslich R, Angus EM, Galle PR, Schneider C, Lammersdorf K, Montrose MH, Neurath MF (2006) Proof of gaps in human small and large intestinal epithelium by in vivo histology with confocal laser endoscopy. Gastroenterology 130:A486–A487

5.   Kiesslich R, Goetz M, Bartsch B, Lammersdorf K, Hoffman A, Schneider C, Vieth M, Stolte M, Galle PR, Neurath MF (2006) Antibody aided confocal laser endomicroscopy allows molecular imaging of colorectal lesions in humans. Gastroenterology 130:A312-A312

9

Future Trends in Confocal Laser Endomicroscopy: Improved Imaging Quality and Immunoendoscopy

Raja Atreya, Markus F. Neurath

Key concepts:

- Immunoendoscopy would open new avenues for gastrointestinal endoscopy.
- Specific fluorescence labelled biomarkers might improve diagnostic algorithms.
- The various indications for immunoendoscopy could include improved diagnosis, prognostic evaluation and pre-therapeutic assessment.

10.1 Introduction

Confocal laser endomicroscopy (CLE) is a powerful new technique that permits subsurface imaging at high resolution during ongoing endoscopy in the upper and lower GI tract [1]. Here, we will discuss future trends in CLE and their potential application in clinical practice. In particular, we will focus on molecular imaging using labelled antibodies for immunoendoscopy.

Recent progress in the field of clinical gastroenterology has led to considerable advances in imaging technologies in gastrointestinal endoscopy. One of the major proceedings in this field consists of the development of endomicroscopic analysis during ongoing endoscopy. The integration of a confocal system into the tip of a conventional video endoscope allows detailed analysis of the mucosa in the GI tract, and this approach emerges as a powerful tool for performing in vivo imaging in mucosal tissue at the cellular and subcellular level. This endoscopic technique incorporates the benefits of high-resolution imaging of confocal microscopy and enables subsequent in situ immunofluorescence staining or other fluorescent labelling techniques. This novel method could change the current practice of clinical gastroenterology as it acquires various potential applications. The possibility to examine mucosal histology during the course of endoscopic procedures is especially beneficial in distinguishing between neoplastic and non-neoplastic tissue, where the subsequent danger of sampling errors of the taken biopsies is inherent. This approach is advantageous in endoscopic surveillance of gastrointestinal disorders such as inflammatory bowel disease or Barrett's oesophagus, in which the mucosa may appear normal when analysed by conventional endoscopy. Apart from its value for diagnosis, the potential benefit of this new technology may extend beyond in vivo histopathology, as this method in combination with in situ immunostaining clearly possesses the potential to further enhance the therapeutic yield of gastrointestinal endoscopy. With the application of various biomarkers (e.g. specific antibodies) this may include investigation of such mucosal processes as inflammation, barrier alterations, atypical migration of cells or clinical monitoring of therapeutic interventions in gastrointestinal disorders.

The following sections provide an overview of the diagnostic and therapeutic potential of antibody applications in vivo and subsequent imaging through endomicroscopic endoscopy. Following a general introduction referring to the basic structure of and differences among antibodies, special emphasis is put on the ongoing efforts to take full advantage of the clinical utility of murine monoclonal antibodies through reduction of their immunogenic properties. Furthermore, newer developments in the field of immunohistology are presented that promise to generate further insights into the pathogenesis of different inflammatory and tumour diseases of the gastrointestinal tract and may enable the staining of target molecules to identify disease entities that can successfully be treated with monoclonal antibodies. This development in endoscopic imaging gives hope for improved diagnosis and targeted therapies in gastrointestinal disorders [1–3].

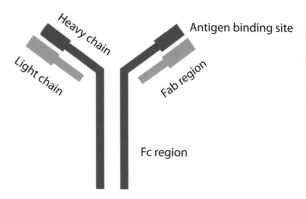

◻ Fig. 10.1. Structure of an antibody

10.2 Characterisation of Antibodies as Diagnostic and Research Instruments

Antibodies are soluble glycoproteins of the immunoglobulin superfamily that all share the same basic structural characteristics but display considerable variability in the regions that bind the antigen. The variability of the antigen-binding regions accounts for the capacity of the antibodies to bind to various antigens. While mammals express five types of antibodies with subsequent subtypes, by far the most commonly used immunoglobulin in immunohistochemistry is immunoglobulin G (IgG). In some cases immunoglobulin M (IgM) is used.

10.2.1 Antibody Structure

The basic unit of each antibody is a »Y«-shaped monomer consisting of four polypeptide chains with two identical heavy and light chains (◻ Fig. 10.1). The heavy chain defines the antibody class. Each heavy chain has a constant region that is the same for all immunoglobulins of the same class and a variable region that is identical for all immunoglobulins produced by a single B cell. The light chains consist mostly of two types, called kappa and lambda, and of two distinct domains: a constant and a variable region. The Fc (fragment crystallisable) region is the tail of the »Y«-shaped antibody and is composed of two heavy chains. This region binds predominantly to various cell receptors and physiologically mediates different effects of antibodies. The bivalent Fab (fragment antigen binding) region is the antigen-binding portion of the antibody and is composed of one constant and one

variable domain each of the heavy and the light chain. The antigen-binding site at the amino terminal end of the antibody is called the paratope, which binds to the tertiary structure of the epitope on the specific antigens through a cascade of non-covalent bonding interactions. The antibody-antigen bond is imparted through a combination of Van der Waals forces and electrostatic interactions.

10.2.2 Diagnostic Monoclonal and Polyclonal Antibodies

In the field of research, antibodies are used mostly to identify intracellular and extracellular proteins. Polyclonal antibodies are generally produced by immunising animals (mouse, rabbits, goats, sheep or horses) with purified antigens. This leads to the production of specific antibodies that bind the antigen and can be extracted from the antiserum of the animal. The polyclonal antisera are commonly purified with protein A/G or antigen affinity chromatography to eliminate irrelevant antibodies.

Monoclonal antibodies are normally produced in mice and rabbits, which are injected with the purified antibody. After the subsequent immune reaction has taken place, the B lymphocytes are extracted from the spleen and are fused with murine myeloma cells. This leads to the formation of a hybrid cell (hybridoma) that produces monoclonal antibodies against a specific epitope. These hybridoma cells are immortal cells that are kept in cell cultures or in the peritoneum of mice.

As polyclonal antisera include various, heterogeneous antibodies against multiple epitopes of the target antigen, they have a higher sensitivity but lower specificity com-

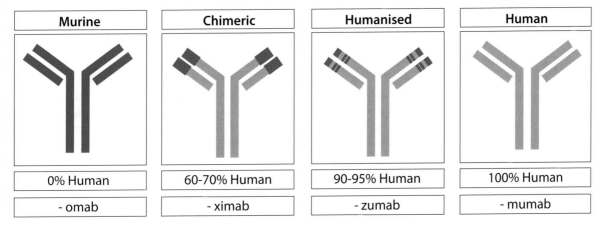

Fig. 10.2. Therapeutic monoclonal antibodies

pared with monoclonal antibodies. Therefore, polyclonal antibodies have a higher potential for detecting an antigen due to their broad range of epitope recognition, but accordingly also possess a higher chance of cross-reactivity with other proteins that have similar epitopes, leading to false-positive results. Monoclonal antibodies, on the other hand, have a high specificity that reduces the possibility of cross-reactivity with other antigens [4, 5].

10.2.3 Therapeutic Monoclonal Antibodies

While the use of monoclonal antibodies in the diagnostic field is well established, they have also been used recently in the therapy of a steadily increasing number of indications and thus have become a major asset in the therapeutic regime of various diseases.

However, initial studies with murine monoclonal antibodies also revealed their limitations in the clinical setting, as rodent monoclonal antibodies in human beings can potentially initiate an immunogenic response, leading to the development of human anti-mouse antibodies (HAMA) [6]. Besides the occurrence of adverse advents, this could also lead to a relatively faster clearance of the antibodies and therefore reduce their therapeutic benefit. Subsequent research activities concentrated on the reduction of the murine content of the therapeutic antibodies. This led to the development of mouse-human chimeric monoclonal antibodies by fusing the murine variable domains to human constant domains (Fig. 10.2). Chimeric antibodies have 60–70% human sequences and several

of them have been approved as therapeutic agents. Infliximab, for instance, is a clinically established chimeric IgG1 antibody against the proinflammatory cytokine TNF-α, used in the treatment of inflammatory bowel disease [7]. As chimeric antibodies still contain murine variable domains, they are potentially immunogenic in patients. Significant reduction of the potential immunogenicity of the murine variable regions was achieved through further humanisation by complementarity-determining region (CDR) grafting, i.e the transfer of the CDR and a few selected framework residues of the mouse variable regions onto human variable region acceptor frameworks. This leads to reduction of the murine content in the sequence of a CDR-grafted antibody by 5–10%. The retention of murine framework residues is crucial for retaining the antigen-binding activity of the antibody, but at the same time potential immunogenicity is also heightened [6]. An approved humanised antibody for clinical use is alemtuzumab, an anti-CD52 antibody used in the treatment of B-cell chronic lymphocytic leukaemia. Further increase of the human portion of the CDR is achieved by grafting only the specificity-determining residues (SDR) within the CDR, the regions directly involved in antigen binding, onto the human frameworks. Therefore, SDR grafting further maximises the human content of the CDR and minimises its potential immunogenicity in clinical use. With the development of phage display technology, mimicking in vivo affinity maturation through enrichment of antibodies as single-chain Fcs or Fabs displayed on the coat of filamentous phage, it is possible to obtain fully human antibodies, to further humanise a murine antibody or to increase the antigen-binding affinity of an existing humanised antibody [6].

In spite of these various efforts to further humanise newly developed antibodies, it is not possible to exclude immunogenic properties of such antibodies in advance. In fact, the currently available fully human antibody adalimumab, which is directed against TNF-α, may induce HAMA response in some patients in spite of excellent efficacy in other patients [8]. Further humanisation methods to reliably produce antibodies that are optimised for low immunogenicity and high antigen affinity are being developed.

10.3   Immunhistochemistry

Immunohistochemistry is a collective term for diverse methods aimed at recognising antigens in situ by means of labelled antibodies. Since the first report, published in 1942, in which antibodies labelled with fluorescein were employed as a specific histochemical stain detecting antigenic material in tissue sections, the diagnostic possibilities in the field of immunohistochemistry have undergone a remarkable development [9]. The method is now an integral part of diagnosis and research in various diseases.

Immunohistochemistry is based on the detection of an antigen by the means of an initial binding reaction of specific antibodies against this antigen. In order to make this immune reaction visible, a labelling agent is conjugated to the primary, secondary or even tertiary antibody. While several kinds of labelling agents have been developed,

those most frequently used are enzymes (e.g. alkaline phosphatase, peroxidase). Conjugation leads to the formation of a coloured precipitate, which is detected under the microscope, revealing the presence and location of the homologous antigen within a cell or tissue preparation. The applications of this approach for immunohistochemistry are numerous and have come to include, besides the obvious function of structural and functional imaging at the cellular level, diagnostic properties, prognostic evaluation and even pre-therapeutic assessments [5].

10.3.1   Direct Immunostaining

In this rather simple immunohistochemical method (◧ Fig. 10.3) a primary antibody is conjugated with a labelling agent as a histochemical stain and then applied to the tissue. The labels most commonly used are fluorochromes, various enzymes and biotin. This one-step process is easy to realise but is sometimes not sensitive enough to detect certain antigens.

10.3.2   Indirect Immunostaining

In order to increase the sensitivity of antibody detection, the method of indirect immunostaining was developed, consisting of two subsequent steps (◧ Fig. 10.3). The first sequence comprises the application of an unlabelled primary antibody directed against the antigen studied, followed by a labelled secondary antibody against the first antibody. The sensitivity of this method is intensi-

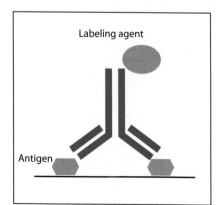
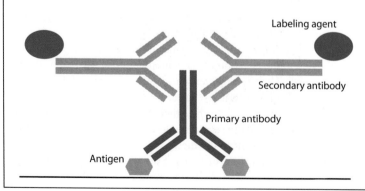

◧ **Fig. 10.3.** Direct and indirect immunostaining

fied through the unlabelled primary antibody, which is unchanged in its activity. Furthermore, at least two or more secondary antibodies are able to bind to each primary antibody, resulting in an amplified signal and the opportunity to detect even smaller amounts of an antibody. A frequently used conjugate is the labelled streptavidin-biotin combination, which consists of a biotinylated secondary antibody and a third reagent of labelled streptavidin. In the presence of the appropriate chromogen, the labelling agent causes the formation of coloured precipitates at the site of the antigen, which can be imaged with conventional light microscopy.

10.3.3 Immunofluorescence

Among the various immunostaining techniques, immunofluorescence has established itself as one of the most

significant and reliable methods of antibody imaging. In this method the fluorochrome labelled antibody is activated through a light source using excitation wavelengths maximally absorbed by the fluorochrome, leading to an immunofluorescence emission that can be quantitatively analysed. The most commonly used labels for fluorescent immunohistochemistry are fluorescein isothiocyanate (FITC) with a green emission or rhodamine conjugates and indocarbocyanine (Cy3) or indodicarbocyanide (Cy5) that emit orange to red fluorescence (◻ Fig. 10.4). The great advantages of fluorescent-labelled substances are their high sensitivity and the linear relationship between the immunofluorescence emission and the detected antigen concentration. Moreover, the use of multiple-band filter sets in the microscope enables the simultaneous visualisation of different fluorescent colours, which is instrumental for in situ verification of antibody co-localization [10].

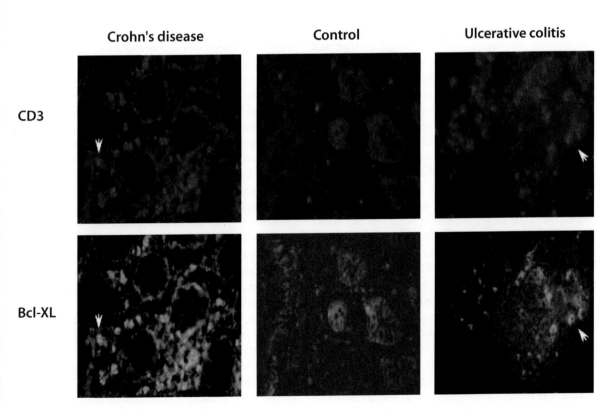

◻ **Fig. 10.4.** Immunohistochemical double-staining analysis of the cellular expression of CD3 and bcl-XL in colonic specimens of IBD patients and controls. *Arrowheads* depict double-positive cells

10.4   In Vivo Fluorescence Endomicroscopy for Immunoendoscopy

The detection of specific proteins by labelled antibodies has previously been restricted to imaging in cell and tissue preparations, but the development of confocal laser endomicroscopy gives hope that these antibodies can also be used for in vivo functional imaging. A further benefit of in vivo immunostaining lies in the possibility for the antigen to retain its immunological activity while the architecture and cytology of the tissue is preserved, enabling more precise examination of the antigen in its »natural« surrounding. Furthermore, the possibility of a non-destructive in situ method to perform mucosal immunostaining, without the risk of physical bleeding while taking a mucosal sample, may reduce the rate of complications.

As confocal laser endomicroscopy enables high-resolution subsurface imaging of living cells in the mucosa during ongoing endoscopy, its use in conjunction with contrast agents that are visualised by the solid-state blue laser integrated in the endoscopic system potentiates the distinctive imaging of cellular structures. The great advantage of confocal imaging lies in its sensitivity to fluorescence, resulting in enhanced image contrast and resolution, revealing sharp cellular and subcellular details. Tissue autofluorescence due to excitation of endogenous tissue fluorophores in collagen or other cellular components has been used to detect neoplasms in the gastrointestinal tract, but overall the inducible fluorescence was too weak to enable sufficient imaging. Therefore, exogenous fluorophores that could be excited by the 488-nm wavelength emitted by the solid-state laser used in confocal endoscopy were used. Initial studies with the intravenous fluorescent contrast agents actraflavine and fluorescein have shown promising results in the detection of malignant mucosa [1]. The extended diagnostic potential of this method has recently also been demonstrated by in vivo diagnosis of *Helicobacter pylori* infection during ongoing gastroscopy, therefore enabling rapid therapy directly after the intervention [11]. The further development and possible in vivo application of new antibodies detecting several different antigens, ranging from proteins to infectious agents and even distinctive subsets of cells, could significantly broaden the therapeutic and diagnostic yield of gastrointestinal endoscopy. In fact, it was recently found that CLE in conjunction with direct immunofluorescence with labelled antibodies was capable of detecting specific markers on epithelial cells in the colonic mucosa (e.g. CD44) ex vivo (R. Kiesslich, M.F. Neurath, unpublished data). The following section provides another example of possible clinical applications of in vivo fluorescence endomicroscopy, elucidating the pathogenic role of certain target molecules that are believed to be involved in disease pathogenesis.

10.4.1   In Vivo Fluorescence Endomicroscopy in Inflammatory Bowel Disease

Inflammatory bowel diseases (IBD) comprise Crohn's disease and ulcerative colitis, which are defined as chronic inflammations of the gastrointestinal tract not due to specific pathogens [12]. Although the precise aetiology of inflammatory bowel disease remains unclear, augmented T-cell resistance to apoptosis is regarded as a pivotal factor in the pathogenesis [13]. While normal intestinal lamina propria T cells are highly susceptible to apoptosis, mucosal lymphocytes in Crohn's disease are less vulnerable to Fas-mediated apoptosis, which corresponds with an increased concentration of the anti-apoptotic protein Bcl-xl [14, 15]. Therefore novel therapeutic strategies aim at restoring intestinal T-cell susceptibility to apoptosis by targeting signal molecules that are pivotal for augmented apoptosis resistance in inflammatory bowel disease. The therapeutic rationale of the well-established treatment with chimeric anti-TNF-α monoclonal antibodies in IBD also seems to lie in rapid and augmented induction of intestinal T-cell apoptosis. However, 30% of patients with refractory Crohn's disease have been found to be resistant against α-TNF therapy. Therefore, it is crucial to find predictors to select suitable patients for treatment beforehand, avoiding futile exposure to the toxicity of this substance [16]. Recent studies indicate that this induction of apoptosis is mediated by outside-to-inside (reverse) signalling through transmembrane TNF-α (mTNF), as its bipolar function enables mTNF to act as a ligand and as a receptor [17]. Therefore, routine endocolonoscopy with fluorescence staining of the mTNF in IBD patients prior to TNF-α treatment could quantify the mTNF expression and might serve as a good predictor for the clinical efficacy of the antibody application in these patients. In such a possible clinical setting immunoendoscopy might be a valuable asset in pre-therapeutic disease assessment. Furthermore, it could also be used in the clinical monitoring after antibody therapy, as pro-apoptotic members of the Bcl-2 family are transcriptionally up-regulated in the intestine after TNF-α therapy [18] and subsequent in vivo immunofluorescence endomicroscopy detecting these proteins could evaluate the clinical response.

10.4.2 In Vivo Fluorescence Endomicroscopy in Cancer Treatment

In recent years, progressive new treatment regimens have evolved around the basic concept of targeting specific molecules expressed by malignant cells, which have an essential role in the regulation of proliferation and growth. Several types of monoclonal antibodies have been produced in the treatment of tumours that express large amounts of these target molecules. Therefore, immuno-histological detection of these biomarkers in the tumour has direct therapeutic consequences, as it enables a subsequent antibody treatment.

Imatinib is a well-established chemotherapeutic agent of kinase-targeted treatment that has found increasing use in cancer treatment. Approximately >90% of gastrointestinal stomal tumours (GIST) express the CD 117 (c-kit) antigen and have mutations in the corresponding gene, and a large majority of GIST patients benefit from treatment with imatinib, which is the main therapeutic modality in this disease. Therefore, in vivo fluorescence endomicroscopy detecting CD 117 in these tumours could be an effective method to identify which patients would benefit from imatinib therapy [19]. Other possible applications for in vivo fluorescence endomicroscopy might be the assessment of the epidermal-growth-factor-receptor (EGFR) expression in therapy-refractory colorectal carcinoma, which could stratify the patient population eligible for cetuximab treatment [20].

10.5 Conclusion

If the technique of in vivo fluorescence endomicroscopy could successfully be adapted to clinical practice and frequently used during examination, it certainly would open new avenues for gastrointestinal endoscopy. Apart from the anticipated development of new specific fluorescence-labelled biomarkers of disease, the awaited future development of greater depths of optical sectioning could enable even more advanced tissue penetration. In addition, modern techniques such as two-photon imaging might result in higher resolution of cell-cell interactions or subcellular

details when successfully adapted to confocal endoscopy systems. The various indications for endoscopic interventions in this setting could include improved diagnosis, prognostic evaluation and pre-therapeutic assessment. Furthermore, this approach may be an attractive tool for in vivo studies of several gastrointestinal disorders such as inflammatory bowel disease or malignant tumours, thereby augmenting our knowledge of disease pathogenesis and allowing individualised therapies.

References

1. Kiesslich R, Burg J, Vieth M, Gnaendiger J, Enders M, Delaney P, Polglase A, McLaren W, Janell D, Thomas S, Nafe B, Galle PR, Neurath MF (2004) Confocal laser endoscopy for diagnosing intraepithelial neoplasias and colorectal cancer in vivo. Gastroenterology 127:706–713
2. Polglase AL, McLaren WJ, Skinner SA, Kiesslich R, Neurath MF, Delaney PM (2005) A fluorescence confocal endomicroscope for in vivo microscopy of the upper- and the lower-GI tract. Gastrointest Endosc 62:686–695
3. Scoazec JY (2003) Tissue and cell imaging in situ: potential for applications in pathology and endoscopy. Gut 52: [Suppl 4]:1–6
4. Abul K. Abbas, Lichtman AHJ (2005) Cellular and molecular immunology. Saunders, Philadelphia, pp 43–50
5. Ramos-Vara JA (2005) Technical aspects of immunohistochemistry. Vet Pathol 42:405–426
6. Gonzales NR, De Pascalis R, Schlom J, Kashmiri SV (2005) Minimizing the immunogenicity of antibodies for clinical application. Tumour Biol 26: 31–43
7. Van Dullemen HM, van Deventer SJ, Hommes DW, Bijl HA., Jansen J, Tytgat GN, Woody J (1995) Treatment of Crohn's disease with anti-tumor necrosis factor chimeric monoclonal antibody (cA2). Gastroenterology 109:129–135
8. Bender NK, Heilig CE, Droll B, Wohlgemuth J, Armbruster FP, Heilig B (2007) Immunogenicity, efficacy and adverse events of adalimumab in RA patients. Rheumatol Int 27:269–274
9. Coons AH, Kaplan MH (1950) Localization of antigen in tissue cells; improvements in a method for the detection of antigen by means of fluorescent antibody. J Exp Med 91:1–13
10. Brandtzaeg P (1998) The increasing power of immunohistochemistry and immunocytochemistry. J Immunol Methods 216:49–67
11. Kiesslich R, Goetz M, Burg J, Stolte M, Siegel E, Maeurer MJ, Thomas S, Strand D, Galle PR, Neurath MF (2005) Diagnosing Helicobacter pylori in vivo by confocal laser endoscopy. Gastroenterology. 128:2119–2123
12. Podolsky DK (1991) Inflammatory bowel disease. N Engl J Med 325:928–937
13. Neurath MF, Finotto S, Fuss I, Boirivant M, Galle PR, Strober W (2001) Regulation of T-cell apoptosis in inflammatory bowel disease: to die or not to die, that is the mucosal question. Trends Immunol 22:21–26
14. Rutgeerts P, van Deventer S, Schreiber S (2003) Review article: the expanding role of biological agents in the treatment of inflamma-

tory bowel disease – focus on selective adhesion molecule inhibition. Aliment Pharmacol Ther 17:1435–1450

15. Ina K, Binion DG, West GA, Dobrea GM, Fiocchi C (1995) Crohn's disease (CD) mucosal T-cells are resistant to apoptosis. Gastroenterology 108:A841

16. Rutgeerts P, Van Assche G, Vermeire S (2004) Optimizing anti-TNF treatment in inflammatory bowel disease. Gastroenterology 126:1593–1610

17. Corazza N, Brunner T, Buri C, Rihs S, Imboden MA, Seibold I, Mueller C (2004) Transmembrane tumor necrosis factor is a potent inducer of colitis even in the absence of its secreted form. Gastroenterology. 127:816–825

18. Lugering A, Schmidt M, Lugering N, Pauels HG, Domschke W, Kucharzik T (2001) Infliximab induces apoptosis in monocytes from patients with chronic active Crohn's disease by using a caspase-dependent pathway. Gastroenterology 121:1145–1157

19. Nowain A, Bhakta H, Pais S, Kanel G, Verma SJ (2005) Gastrointestinal stromal tumors: clinical profile, pathogenesis, treatment strategies and prognosis. Gastroenterol Hepatol 20: 818–824

20. Goldstein NS, Armin M (2001) Epidermal growth factor receptor immunohistochemical reactivity in patients with American Joint Committee on Cancer Stage IV colon adenocarcinoma: implications for a standardized scoring system. Cancer 92:1331–1346

10

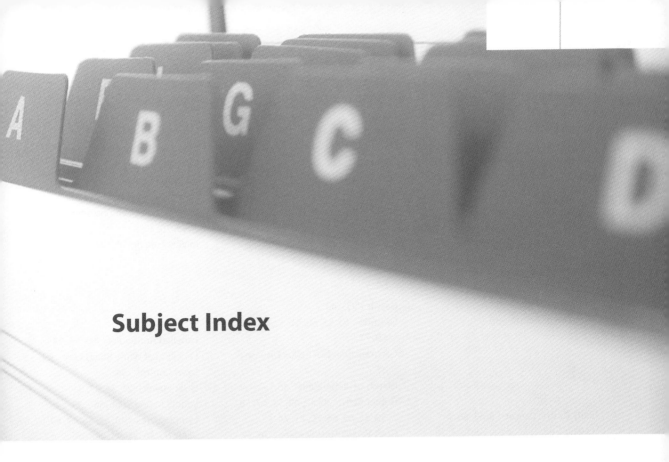

Subject Index